BMA

Get Ahead!
Basic
Sciences
500 SBAs

Priya Jeevananthan
Obstetric and Gynaecology Registrar
Queen Charlotte's and Chelsea Hospital, London

Anna Kowalewski
Foundation Doctor, London

Series Editor
Saran Shantikumar
Academic Clinical Fellow in Public Health
University of Warwick
Coventry, UK

CRC Press
Taylor & Francis Group
Boca Raton London New York

CRC Press is an imprint of the
Taylor & Francis Group, an **informa** business

D0313853

CRC Press
Taylor & Francis Group
6000 Broken Sound Parkway NW, Suite 300
Boca Raton, FL 33487-2742

Printed in Great Britain by Ashford Colour Press Ltd
Version Date: 20161017

International Standard Book Number-13: 978-1-4987-5098-1 (Paperback)

**Visit the Taylor & Francis Web site at
http://www.taylorandfrancis.com**

**and the CRC Press Web site at
http://www.crcpress.com**

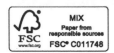

Contents

Preface   v
Contributors   vii

Questions Paper 1   1

Answers Paper 1   11

Questions Paper 2   21

Answers Paper 2   31

Questions Paper 3   41

Answers Paper 3   51

Questions Paper 4   59

Answers Paper 4   69

Questions Paper 5   79

Answers Paper 5   89

Questions Paper 6   97

Answers Paper 6   107

Questions Paper 7   117

Answers Paper 7   127

Questions Paper 8   137

Answers Paper 8   147

Questions Paper 9   157

Answers Paper 9   167

Questions Paper 10   179

Answers Paper 10   189

Index   199

Preface

Welcome to *Get Ahead! Basic Sciences: 500 SBAs*.

The book contains a collection of SBAs to help you practice for your Basic Sciences exam, covering topics in anatomy, physiology, pharmacology and biochemistry. In addition to testing core knowledge, the questions also encompass important problems that are relevant to clinical practice.

Practice questions are the best way of reinforcing knowledge and give you a realistic idea of how effective your revision is. As you draw closer to your exam, it is important to do as many practice questions as you can in order to familiarize yourself with the thought process and to do whole practice papers so you pace yourself correctly on the actual day of the exam. The more questions you do, the more you will begin to see the common themes and patterns that are easy marks to pick up in the exam, which can be the difference between a pass and a fail.

We have divided this book into 10 papers, each consisting of 50 questions with detailed answers supplied at the end of each paper. Explanations have been provided to help you understand the right answer and why the other options are not correct. You should aim to take 60 minutes on each paper, leaving you around a minute for each question.

We hope this book, and its companion volume *Get Ahead! Basic Sciences: 100 EMQs*, helps you prepare, and most importantly pass, your exams! Best of luck to you and remember to practice, practice, practice!

Priya Jeevananthan
Anna Kowalewski

Contributors

WRITTEN AND EDITED BY
Priya Jeevananthan
Anna Kowalewski

ADDITIONAL CONTRIBUTORS
Neel Sharma
Avishek Das
Daniel Glassman
Pavithra Logitharajah
Chinedu Maduakor
Vikram Malhotra
Ian Mann
John Nehme
Naomi Periselmeris
Donna Pilkington
James Richardson
Ravnita Sharma
Naren Srinivasan
Stephanie Stone
Helen Butler

SERIES EDITOR
Saran Shantikumar

Questions Paper 1

1. The Edinger–Westphal nucleus is associated with which of the following cranial nerves?
   A. CN III
   B. CN IV
   C. CN VII
   D. CN IX
   E. CN X

2. Which of the following causes an increased anion gap?
   A. Diabetic ketoacidosis
   B. Diarrhoea
   C. Hyperventilation
   D. Hypoventilation
   E. Vomiting

3. Which of the following muscles are *not* used in respiration?
   A. Diaphragm
   B. Intercostal muscles
   C. Pectoral muscles
   D. Scalene muscles
   E. Sternocleidomastoid muscles

4. What are the caudate nucleus, putamen and globus pallidus collectively known as?
   A. Basal ganglia
   B. Cerebellum
   C. Diencephalon
   D. Frontal lobe
   E. Neostriatum

5. Within which lobe of the brain is the primary auditory cortex situated?
   A. Frontal
   B. Frontoparietal
   C. Occipital
   D. Parietal
   E. Temporal

6. What lies within the sella turcica of the sphenoid bone?
   A. Amygdala
   B. Cerebellar peduncle

C. Mammillary bodies
D. Pituitary gland
E. Pons

7. Which of the following drains directly into the portal vein?
   A. Left and right gastric veins
   B. Left gastroepiploic vein
   C. Right gastroepiploic vein
   D. All of the options A to C
   E. None of the options A to C

8. Pyruvate is converted via pyruvate carboxylase to what?
   A. Acetyl-CoA
   B. Citrate
   C. Oxaloacetate
   D. Oxoglutarate
   E. Succinate

9. Which one of the following statements regarding haemoglobin metabo-lism in humans is *not* true?
   A. Ageing or damaged red blood cells are removed from the circulation by macrophages of the spleen, liver and bone marrow.
   B. Bilirubin is bound to glucuronic acid in the liver and kidney by the enzyme glucuronyl transferase.
   C. Conjugated bilirubin is excreted in bile and enters the small intestine.
   D. Globin is separated from haem and then converted to bilirubin.
   E. If there is increased red cell turnover, bilirubin and urobilinogen excretion increases.

10. Severe vomiting will lead to which acid–base disturbance?
    A. Metabolic acidosis
    B. Metabolic alkalosis
    C. No disturbance
    D. Respiratory acidosis
    E. Respiratory alkalosis

11. Carbimazole is within which class of drugs?
    A. β-Adrenoceptor antagonists
    B. Glucocorticoids
    C. Iodides
    D. Radioiodine
    E. Thioureylenes

12. Which biochemical marker is most commonly raised in rhabdomyolysis and muscular dystrophy?
    A. Alanine aminotransferase
    B. Amylase
    C. Bence Jones proteins

D. Creatinine

E. Creatine phosphokinase

13. Which of the following terminates the activity of noradrenaline at the synaptic cleft?

A. Acetylcholinesterase

B. Catechol-O-methyltransferase

C. Dopa-decarboxylase

D. Glutamate carboxypeptidase II

E. Lipase

14. Which muscle is the antagonist of elbow flexion?

A. Biceps brachii

B. Brachialis

C. Pronator teres

D. Trapezius

E. Triceps brachii

15. The accommodation reflex of the eye is regulated by the autonomic nervous control of which of the following muscles?

A. Ciliary muscle of the eye

B. Inferior oblique muscle of the eye

C. Müller muscles

D. Orbicularis oculi muscles

E. Superior oblique muscle of the eye

16. Preganglionic neurons of the sympathetic division that innervate the stomach, liver and small intestine pass through which of the following ganglia?

A. Coeliac ganglion

B. Inferior mesenteric ganglion

C. Pelvic ganglion

D. Superior cervical ganglion

E. Superior mesenteric ganglion

17. Which of the following is *not* a type of white blood cell?

A. Basophil

B. Eosinophil

C. Monocyte

D. Polymorphonuclear neutrophil

E. Thrombocyte

18. How much energy is contained in a phosphate-to-phosphate bond in a molecule of adenosine triphosphate?

A. 14.2 kJ/mol

B. 18.2 kJ/mol

C. 30.5 kJ/mol

D. 40.5 kJ/mol

E. 45.5 kJ/mol

19. Noradrenaline acts on cardiac muscle to stimulate heart rate and force of contraction via which of the following receptors?
    A. α-Adrenergic receptors
    B. α2-Adrenergic receptors
    C. β-Adrenergic receptors
    D. Both β- and α-adrenergic receptors
    E. None of the above

20. Which muscle is supplied by the long thoracic nerve to rotate the scapula?
    A. Deltoid
    B. Latissimus dorsi
    C. Levator scapulae
    D. Serratus anterior
    E. Teres major

21. Within which layer of the gastrointestinal tract is Auerbach's plexus found?
    A. Lamina propria
    B. Muscularis externa
    C. Muscularis mucosa
    D. Serosa
    E. Submucosa

22. Caseous necrosis can be seen histologically in which of the following conditions?
    A. Ankylosing spondylitis
    B. Colonic carcinoma
    C. Hepatitis
    D. Lupus glomerulonephritis
    E. Tuberculosis

23. Which of the following is a common cause of necrotizing fasciitis?
    A. *Corynebacterium* sp.
    B. *Listeria monocytogenes*
    C. *Mycobacterium* sp.
    D. *Nocardia asteroides*
    E. *Streptococcus pyogenes*

24. Bronchoconstriction of the bronchial tree is caused by which of the following?
    A. Parasympathetic innervation via the phrenic nerve
    B. Parasympathetic innervation via T3–T6
    C. Parasympathetic innervation via the vagus nerve
    D. Sympathetic innervation via T3–T6
    E. Sympathetic innervation via the vagus nerve

25. Angiotensin II receptor antagonists are contraindicated in which of the following patients?
    A. Patients already on an angiotensin-converting enzyme inhibitor
    B. Patients on potassium-sparing diuretics
    C. Patients who suffered a cough with ramipril
    D. Patients with bilateral renal artery stenosis
    E. Patients with microalbuminuria

26. Which one of the following statements regarding oxygen transport and haemoglobin is *false*?
    A. A single haemoglobin molecule can carry up to four molecules of oxygen.
    B. Each haemoglobin molecule contains four globin chains and four haem units, each with four atoms of iron.
    C. Haemoglobin binds reversibly to oxygen to form oxyhaemoglobin.
    D. Haemoglobin contains globin and a pigmented iron-containing complex.
    E. In the lungs oxyhaemoglobin formation is favoured to dissociation.

27. Which of the following options regarding the aetiology of polycystic kidney disease is correct?
    A. Autoimmune: anti-glomerular basement membrane (anti-GBM) antibodies
    B. Genetic: autosomal dominant
    C. Genetic: X-linked recessive
    D. Infective: schistosomiasis
    E. Inflammatory: drug-induced

28. Which of the following is *incorrect* with regard to necrosis?
    A. Cells swell in size.
    B. It affects large groups of cells.
    C. It is an inflammatory response.
    D. It is caused by irreversible injury.
    E. There is peripheral condensation of chromatin.

29. Which one of the following medications is used in benign prostatic hyperplasia to reduce prostate size by inhibiting the metabolism of testosterone?
    A. Doxazosin
    B. Finasteride
    C. Metoprolol
    D. Spironolactone
    E. Tamsulosin

30. Which of the following best describes the action of the muscle relaxant suxamethonium?
    A. It blocks calcium ion channels at the neuromuscular junction.
    B. It can be reversed by anticholinesterases.

C. It is a non-depolarizing neuromuscular blocker.
D. It is an acetylcholinesterase inhibitor.
E. It mimics acetylcholine at the neuromuscular junctions.

31. Which of the following is a drug used to improve the symptoms of myasthenia gravis?
    A. Atenolol
    B. Baclofen
    C. Mirtazapine
    D. Pyridostigmine
    E. Suxamethonium

32. Parasympathetic innervation to the heart reduces the force of contraction via which nerve?
    A. Accessory nerve
    B. Glossopharyngeal nerve
    C. Intercostal nerves
    D. Phrenic nerve
    E. Vagus nerve

33. Which of the following is most appropriate for the treatment of nocturnal leg cramps?
    A. Co-proxamol
    B. Morphine
    C. Oramorph
    D. Paracetamol
    E. Quinine

34. Which of the following anticoagulants can be monitored by measuring the activated partial thrombin time?
    A. Aspirin
    B. Clopidogrel
    C. Dipyridamole
    D. Heparin
    E. Warfarin

35. During the conversion of malate to oxaloacetate in the Krebs cycle, a molecule of what is formed?
    A. CO_2
    B. GTP
    C. H_2
    D. H_2O
    E. NADH

36. Which of the following is *incorrect* with regard to apoptosis?
    A. Cells shrink to form apoptotic bodies.
    B. It can be triggered by DNA damage.

C. It is also known as programmed cell death.
D. It is associated with specific gene activation.
E. It usually affects large groups of cells.

37. With regard to the ABO system of blood grouping, which one of the following is *incorrect*?
A. Blood group A, as a donor, is incompatible with only blood group B.
B. Blood group AB, as a donor, is incompatible with A, B and O.
C. Blood group AB is the universal recipient.
D. Blood group B, as a donor, is compatible with B and AB.
E. Blood group O is the universal donor.

38. Which of the following drugs does flumazenil reverse?
A. Atracurium
B. Atropine
C. Diazepam
D. Methadone
E. Morphine

39. Malignant hyperpyrexia is precipitated by which of the following agents?
A. Diazepam
B. Prilocaine
C. Propofol
D. Suxamethonium
E. Thiopental

40. Which of the following organisms is *not* usually found in the sputum of a patient with cystic fibrosis?
A. *Burkholderia cepacia*
B. *Haemophilus influenzae*
C. *Legionella pneumophila*
D. *Pseudomonas aeruginosa*
E. *Staphylococcus aureus*

41. On which chromosome is the gene for the defective protein for the cystic fibrosis transmembrane conductance regulator coded?
A. Chromosome 7
B. Chromosome 8
C. Chromosome 9
D. Chromosome 10
E. Chromosome 11

42. Which of the following is a sign of digoxin toxicity?
A. Blurred vision and xanthopsia
B. Gynaecomastia
C. Hypokalaemia
D. Hypercalcaemia
E. Reversed tick pattern on the electrocardiogram

43. From which type of cell does a carcinoid tumour develop?
    A. Enterocyte
    B. Enteroendocrine cells
    C. Goblet cells
    D. Paneth cells
    E. Stem cells

44. Which of the following provides arterial supply to the lesser curvature of the stomach?
    A. Left gastric artery
    B. Left gastroepiploic artery
    C. Right and left gastric arteries
    D. Right gastric artery
    E. Right gastroepiploic artery

45. Which of the following dysfunctional tumour suppressor genes is involved in colorectal cancer?
    A. *APC*
    B. *BRCA1*
    C. *NF1*
    D. *p53*
    E. *RB1*

46. Which of the following drugs may cause a dry cough?
    A. Angiotensin II receptor antagonists
    B. Angiotensin-converting enzyme inhibitors
    C. β-Blockers
    D. Calcium channel blockers
    E. Potassium channel blockers

47. Which of the following best describes the pathogenesis of myasthenia gravis?
    A. A defect in the myosin filaments of skeletal muscle
    B. Demyelination of motor neurons
    C. Destruction of the neuromuscular junction by demyelinating disease
    D. Presence of autoantibodies against the acetylcholine receptors at the neuromuscular junction
    E. Reduced number of motor end-plates

48. Which of the following is *not* associated with irreversible cell injury?
    A. Cell death
    B. Dense body formation within mitochondria
    C. Dissociation of ribosomes
    D. Nuclear degeneration
    E. Release of cellular enzymes

49. Which of the following dysfunctional tumour suppressor genes is involved in ovarian cancer?
    A. *APC*
    B. *BRCA1*
    C. *NF1*
    D. *p53*
    E. *RB1*

50. Which of the following is indicated for the treatment of neuropathic pain?
    A. Amitriptyline
    B. Baclofen
    C. Co-proxamol
    D. Diclofenac
    E. Paracetamol

Answers Paper 1

1. A – CN III

Oculomotor, facial, glossopharyngeal and vagus nerves have axons that originate from preganglionic neurons, which synapse at their respective terminal ganglia. Oculomotor (CN III) preganglionic parasympathetic neurons originate from the Edinger–Westphal nucleus and end in the ciliary ganglion. Postganglionic neurons travel in short ciliary nerves to supply the sphincter pupillae muscle of the iris (which causes pupil constriction) and the ciliary muscles (which change the shape of the lens). These play a key role in the pupillary light reflex and accommodation.

2. A – Diabetic ketoacidosis

The anion gap is the difference between the measured cations (Na^+ and K^+) and anions (chloride and bicarbonate). The pathological presence of additional unmeasured anions, with a concurrent reduction in chloride or bicarbonate concentrations, will result in an increased anion gap. For example, in diabetic ketoacidosis, water-soluble ketones are produced as a by-product of fatty acid metabolism. Ketones are also anions and will be buffered by a reduction in bicarbonate, thus resulting in an increased anion gap. The other conditions listed will cause some degree of metabolic disturbance but will not increase the anion gap.

3. C – Pectoral muscles

The principal muscles of respiration include the diaphragm and the intercostal muscles. The diaphragm contracts, enlarging the thoracic cavity and decreasing intrathoracic pressure. This draws air into the lungs via the pressure gradient. As the diaphragm relaxes, the inherent elastic recoil of lung tissue pushes air out. The external intercostals contract during inspiration while the internal and innermost intercostals have a role to play in forced expiration. The scalene and sternocleidomastoid muscles are considered 'accessory' muscles which are used during forced breathing or in pathological states. The pectoral group of muscles are not typically classed as respiratory or accessory muscles.

4. A – Basal ganglia

The caudate nucleus, putamen and globus pallidus are anatomically and functionally closely related, and are collectively known as the basal ganglia. They are responsible for posture and movement.

5. E – Temporal

The primary auditory cortex is found within the superior temporal gyrus of the temporal lobe. The majority of the functional zone is in the superior bank of the gyrus and it is normally hidden within the lateral fissure. There is a small transverse temporal gyrus (or Heschl's convolution) which is an indication of the precise site of the auditory cortex.

6. D – Pituitary gland

The pituitary gland lies within the sella turcica and consists of two cytologically different parts, which are the posterior pituitary (neurohypophysis) and the anterior pituitary (adenohypophysis). The pituitary gland is held by the pituitary stalk, or infundibulum, and lies caudal to the optic chiasm. If the pituitary becomes flattened or shrinks, for instance due to intracranial hypertension or pituitary pathology, it no longer occupies the sella turcica. This is known as *empty sella syndrome.*

7. A – Left and right gastric veins

Only the left and right gastric veins directly drain into the portal vein. The right and left gastroepiploic veins drain into the portal vein indirectly via the superior mesenteric vein and the splenic vein, respectively.

8. C – Oxaloacetate

Pyruvate is metabolized by pyruvate dehydrogenase to form acetyl-CoA. Pyruvate can also be converted by pyruvate carboxylase to oxaloacetate, which is an important intermediary in the tricyclic acid (TCA) cycle. Acetyl-CoA is a two-carbon compound that binds with the four-carbon oxaloacetate to form citrate – a reaction that is catalysed by citrate synthase. Citrate is then converted to an intermediate *cis*-aconitate (via the enzyme aconitase) by removing a water molecule. *cis*-Aconitate is further metabolized by the aconitase and is converted to isocitrate by adding a water molecule. Isocitrate is still a six-carbon compound but it has been structurally altered by the removal and addition of a water molecule. The six-carbon molecule of isocitrate is catalysed by the enzyme isocitrate dehydrogenase to form the five-carbon compound oxoglutarate. During the conversion of isocitrate to oxoglutarate, one molecule of NADH and one molecule of CO_2 are formed.

9. B – Bilirubin is bound to glucuronic acid in the liver and kidney by the enzyme glucuronyl transferase

Glucuronyl transferase is found in the liver (but not in the kidney). This enzyme thus binds bilirubin to glucuronic acid in the liver only.

10. B – Metabolic alkalosis

Severe vomiting leads to the loss of hydrogen ions and other electrolytes. This can result in a metabolic alkalosis for two reasons: firstly through the direct loss of hydrogen ions, and secondly through the increased reabsorption of potassium ions in the kidney, at the expense of hydrogen, to address the electrolyte imbalance.

11. E – Thioureylenes

Both carbimazole and propylthiouracil are thioureylenes. Thioureylenes are used in the treatment of hyperthyroidism. They are thought to act by inhibiting tyrosine residue iodination on thyroglobulin, thus reducing thyroid hormone synthesis.

12. E – Creatine phosphokinase

Creatine phosphokinase is used as a marker of muscle damage. This enzyme catalyses the reaction of creatine and ATP to phosphocreatine and ADP. Phosphocreatine acts as an intramuscular energy store. Circulating creatine phosphokinase levels are elevated in rhabdomyolysis (breakdown of skeletal muscle) and muscular dystrophy, as well as in post-myocardial infarction states, myocarditis and myositis.

13. B – Catechol-O-methyltransferase

Catechol-O-methyltransferase (COMT) is one of several enzymes responsible for degrading the catecholamines noradrenaline and adrenaline. This enzyme is intracellular and found in the postsynaptic neurons. COMT inhibitors are used commonly in the treatment of Parkinson disease, where they prevent the breakdown of therapeutic levodopa by COMT.

14. E – Triceps brachii

In this context, an antagonist is a muscle that opposes a specific movement. Elbow flexion is brought about by contraction of brachialis and biceps brachii. Triceps brachii is the antagonist and contraction results in the opposite movement (i.e. elbow extension). The anconeus muscle also assists with elbow extension, although its relative contribution to this action is trivial. When one muscle in the agonist–antagonist pair is contracted, the other is relaxed, and vice versa.

15. A – Ciliary muscle of the eye

Accommodation is the ability for the eyes to focus upon a nearby object via convergence of the optic axes. This involves contraction of the ciliary muscles which results in an increased convexity of the lens. The accommodation reflex, which is under the control of the Edinger–Westphal nucleus, combines accommodation and convergence with pupil constriction (miosis). While pupillary convergence is necessary to prevent diplopia, the functional requirement for miosis is unknown.

16. A – Coeliac ganglion

The coeliac ganglia are part of the sympathetic prevertebral chain and contribute to the coeliac plexus. The coeliac plexus is the largest nerve plexus and surrounds the coeliac trunk, superior mesenteric arteries and renal arteries at their origin. It is located at the level of T12 and L1. Secondary plexuses branching out from, or connected to, the coeliac plexus are distributed to the upper abdominal organs (e.g. liver, gallbladder, stomach, spleen, pancreas, small bowel and proximal two-thirds of the large bowel).

The coeliac plexus is also known as the *solar plexus* due to the spicule-like radiation of its nerve fibres.

17. E – Thrombocyte

Basophils, monocytes, eosinophils and polymorphonuclear neutrophils are all different types of white blood cell and play a part in infection and the immune system. Thrombocytes are not white blood cells – they are platelets, which are involved in the regulation of blood clotting.

18. C – 30.5 kJ/mol

In cells, reactions that directly produce and consume energy are not linked. Therefore it is necessary to have a short-term method of storing energy within the cells. The molecule adenosine triphosphate (ATP) is the universal energy store. ATP is made up of adenine and a ribose sugar group, which together form adenosine, and three phosphate groups. The energy stored in the phosphate-to-phosphate bond is high at 30.5 kJ/mol. However, the energy stored in the sugar-to-phosphate bond in adenosine monophosphate (AMP) is much lower at 14.2 kJ/mol, which is why it is not used as an energy source for metabolic reactions.

19. C – β-Adrenergic receptors

Increased sympathetic stimulation promotes catecholamine secretion (noradrenaline and adrenaline) by the adrenal medulla, resulting in an increased heart rate and force of contraction, and peripheral vasoconstriction. Noradrenaline acts on β-adrenergic receptors in the heart. This explains the use of β-blockers, such as atenolol, in slowing the heart rate.

20. D – Serratus anterior

Serratus anterior is supplied by the long thoracic nerve (C5–C7). Damage to the long thoracic nerve, which can occur during axillary surgery, results in winging of the scapula. A winged scapula can be demonstrated by asking the patient to push against a wall with both arms.

21. B – Muscularis externa

Auerbach's plexus is part of the enteric nervous system. It is found between the longitudinal and circular layers of the muscularis externa. It provides both sympathetic and parasympathetic input to the gastrointestinal tract.

22. E – Tuberculosis

Mycobacterium tuberculosis is an acid-fast bacillus which causes tuberculosis. Its granulomatous lesions consist of Langhans giant cells with a central area of caseous necrosis. Caseous necrosis is so named due to its apparent soft and white 'cheese-like' appearance. It can also be seen with syphilis, histoplasmosis and *Cryptococcus* infections.

23. E – *Streptococcus pyogenes*

Necrotizing fasciitis is a subcutaneous infection most commonly caused by β-haemolytic streptococcus (e.g. *Streptococcus pyogenes*). However, methicillin-resistant *Staphylococcus aureus* (MRSA), *Clostridium perfringens* and *Bacteroides fragilis* can also cause this destructive, life-threatening infection. Necrotizing fasciitis is a fulminant deep infection with a high mortality rate. It spreads rapidly, causing massive tissue destruction. Urgent debridement, fasciotomy and aggressive antibiotic treatment are required.

24. C – Parasympathetic innervation via the vagus nerve
Vagal parasympathetic neurons originate from the dorsal motor nucleus of the vagus, which is situated in the medulla underneath the floor of the fourth ventricle. From here they travel to the cardiovascular, respiratory and gastrointestinal systems. In the respiratory system, they cause bronchoconstriction of the bronchial tree.

25. D – Patients with bilateral renal artery stenosis
Patients with bilateral renal artery stenosis become dependent on the renin–angiotensin–aldosterone system in order to maintain renal perfusion. If either an angiotensin-converting enzyme (ACE) inhibitor or angiotensin-receptor blocker (ARB) is employed in the treatment of their hypertension, you will essentially complete a chemical nephrectomy. ACE inhibitors and ARBs can be used together, under strict guidance, for the treatment of heart failure and also hypertension.

26. B – Each haemoglobin molecule contains four globin chains and four haem units, each with four atoms of iron
Each haemoglobin molecule contains four globin chains and four haem units, each with one atom of iron. When oxygen levels are low, oxyhaemoglobin breaks down liberating oxygen to the tissues. When oxygen levels are high, as they are in the lungs, oxyhaemoglobin formation is favoured.

27. B – Genetic: autosomal dominant
Polycystic kidney disease (PKD) is the most common inherited nephropathy in the Western world and is largely inherited in an autosomal dominant fashion. It is characterized by the presence of multiple renal cysts and leads to progressive renal failure. Acute episodes can occur and present with haematuria and loin pain. Associated pathologies include hypertension, subarachnoid haemorrhage (owing to rupture of berry aneurysms), hepatic cysts and renal calculi. Autosomal recessive PCKD is far less common and more clinically serious, with underdeveloped kidneys and a 30% death rate in newborns.

28. E – There is peripheral condensation of chromatin
Necrosis is the premature death of cells secondary to external factors, such as hypoxia, infection or trauma. It tends to affect clusters of cells which are exposed to the same trigger, and is associated with an inflammatory response. Peripheral condensation of chromatin is a feature of apoptosis.

29. B – Finasteride

Benign prostatic hyperplasia (BPH) is a non-malignant increase in prostate size, which is common in older men. About 25–50% of men aged over 65 will have some degree of symptomatic BPH. Symptoms are grouped under the umbrella term 'prostatism' and are a direct result of urinary outlet obstruction. They include hesitancy, poor stream, terminal dribbling and frequency. Drug treatments most commonly used are α-adrenergic blockers (e.g. doxazosin and tamsulosin) and 5α-reductase inhibitors (e.g. finasteride). The former acts as smooth muscle relaxants, relieving obstructive symptoms, and the latter inhibits prostatic testosterone metabolism, thus reducing prostate size.

30. E – It mimics acetylcholine at the neuromuscular junctions

Suxamethonium is a depolarizing neuromuscular blocker. It has a rapid onset and short duration of action, and so is used for short-term paralysis before surgery to allow intubation. Respiration must be assisted or controlled when using neuromuscular blockers. Suxamethonium acts by mimicking acetylcholine at the neuromuscular junction (NMJ), thus resulting in neuromuscular blockade by competitive antagonism. Unlike the non-depolarizing neuromuscular blockers, the actions of suxamethonium cannot be reversed with acetylcholinesterase inhibitors; in fact they potentiate the blockade. Recovery from suxamethonium is spontaneous.

31. D – Pyridostigmine

Myasthenia gravis is an autoimmune disorder in which autoantibodies block acetylcholine (ACh) receptors on the post-synaptic membrane of the neuromuscular junction (NMJ). This results in muscle fatigability, which can be shown as a decrement in evoked muscle potential on repetitive motor neuron stimulation. The extraocular muscles are frequently affected, resulting in diplopia and ptosis in addition to bulbar and proximal muscle involvement. About 90% of patients have some degree of thymic involvement, such as hyperplasia or a thymoma, and thymectomy is an effective treatment in some cases. Medical treatment is with acetylcholinesterase inhibitors (e.g. pyridostigmine or physostigmine), which inhibit ACh metabolism and thus increase its availability for transmission at the NMJ.

32. E – Vagus nerve

The parasympathetic division of the autonomic nervous system does not exhibit a 'flight or fight' response; indeed, it results in a 'rest or digest' response. The vagus nerve provides parasympathetic innervation to the heart where it results in negative inotropic and negative chronotropic effects (i.e. it decreases the force of contraction and the heart rate).

33. E – Quinine

Quinine salts are effective at reducing the frequency of nocturnal leg cramps by about 25% in ambulatory patients. It takes up to 4 weeks before any discernible improvement is noted. Treatment should be interrupted every 3 months to assess whether there is a continued need for quinine treatment. Quinine was primarily used in the treatment of malaria, although it is no longer the first-line therapy.

34. D – Heparin
Heparin is a relatively short-acting intravenous anticoagulant. It has one major beneficial property over other anticoagulants in that reversal of its effects can be easily and rapidly achieved. The major problem with heparin is the requirement to regularly check the activated partial thromboplastin time (APTT) to ensure therapeutic anticoagulation is being achieved. APTT is a measure of the intrinsic coagulation system.

35. E – NADH
Fumarate is a four-carbon compound and it is an intermediary molecule in the citric acid (Krebs) cycle. Fumarate is metabolized by the enzyme fumarate hydratase to form the four-carbon compound malate. During this reaction, a single water molecule is required. Malate is metabolized by the enzyme malate dehydrogenase, which converts malate to oxaloacetate. During the conversion of malate to oxaloacetate, a molecule of NADH is formed. Oxaloacetate is a four-carbon compound and is combined with acetyl-CoA via the enzyme citrate synthase to form the six-carbon compound citrate.

36. E – It usually affects large groups of cells
Apoptosis is programmed cell death, where a sequence of events results in cellular changes with the eventual result of cell death. There may be an underlying increase in the expression of pro-apoptotic genes within the cell. Apoptosis usually affects single cells in contrast to necrosis, which usually affects clusters of cells.

37. A – Blood group A, as a donor, is incompatible with only blood group B
Blood group A, as a donor, is incompatible with B and O, because both make anti-A antibodies that will react with A antigens.

38. C – Diazepam
Flumazenil reverses the effects of benzodiazepines, such as diazepam, by acting as a competitive antagonist. It is an imidazobenzodiazepine and bears a close resemblance to the structure of midazolam. It has a half-life of approximately 50 minutes and is metabolized to a carboxylic acid derivative and glucuronide.

39. D – Suxamethonium
Malignant hyperpyrexia is a myopathic disorder that is characterized by a marked increase in metabolic rate. It is an autosomal dominant condition that can be precipitated by suxamethonium and volatile anaesthetic agents. These agents trigger an abnormal release of calcium from the sarcoplasmic reticulum into the cytoplasm. Symptoms include a rapid rise in temperature, progressive tachycardia, muscle rigidity and masseter spasm.

40. C – *Legionella pneumophila*
Legionella pneumophila is the Gram-negative bacterium responsible for Legionnaires' disease and is not usually found in the sputum of cystic fibrosis patients. Patients with cystic fibrosis are commonly colonized with *Haemophilus* and *Streptococcus* in their early years but are subsequently colonized particularly with *Pseudomonas* and almost invariably with *Burkholderia*.

41. A – Chromosome 7
The defective protein gene is present on the long (q) arm of chromosome 7. It codes for the cystic fibrosis transmembrane conductance regulator (CFTR) – a cyclic adenosine monophosphate (cAMP) regulated chlorine channel which leads to a high concentration of sodium and a low concentration of chloride in exocrine secretions. There are many variants of this defect. The most common mutation is the ΔF508: 'Δ' means a deletion, specifically in this case, of the three nucleotides coding for phenylalanine (F) at position 508 of the gene. This accounts for up to 70% of all mutations.

42. A – Blurred vision and xanthopsia
A reversed tick pattern on an ECG (downward-sloping ST segments) is not a sign of digoxin toxicity, but a sign of digoxin treatment. Gynaecomastia is a relatively common side-effect of long-term treatment, but not of toxicity. Both hypercalcaemia and hypokalaemia predispose patients to developing digoxin toxicity but are not in themselves a result of the toxicity. Blurring of the vision and xanthopsia (yellow vision) can occur in toxicity.

43. B – Enteroendocrine cells
Carcinoid tumours are slow-growing neuroendocrine tumours. Two-thirds of carcinoid tumours are found within the gastrointestinal tract, with the midgut (duodenum to transverse colon) being the location of the primary tumour in up to 75% of gastrointestinal cases. The most notable secretion is serotonin which may cause flushing, diarrhoea, wheezing, abdominal cramping and peripheral oedema.

44. C – Right and left gastric arteries
The left and right gastric arteries supply the lesser curvature of the stomach. They branch from the coeliac trunk via the common hepatic arteries. The right gastroepiploic artery supplies the right side of the greater curvature. It is a branch of the gastroduodenal artery. The left gastroepiploic artery supplies the middle part of the greater curvature and is derived from the splenic artery and ultimately from the coeliac trunk. The short gastric arteries supply the upper part of the greater curvature.

45. A – *APC*
The *APC* (adenomatous polyposis coli) tumour suppressor gene has been implicated in colorectal cancer. It is inherited in an autosomal dominant fashion and is located on the long (q) arm of chromosome 5. Inheritance

results in the presence of between 100 and 1000 tubular adenomas which carpet the colon, and less frequently the stomach and the small bowel (particularly the duodenum). The polyps usually appear in the second and third decade of life and have a 100% malignant potential.

46. B – Angiotensin-converting enzyme inhibitors
ACE (angiotensin-converting enzyme) inhibitors, a commonly used class of antihypertensive, can cause a dry cough due to increases in bradykinin levels secondary to inhibition of degradation. Bradykinin causes blood vessels to dilate and thus lowers the blood pressure, but bradykinin-induced bronchoconstriction may be the cause of the cough seen in some patients.

47. D – Presence of autoantibodies against the acetylcholine receptors at the neuromuscular junction
Myasthenia gravis is an autoimmune condition characterized by the presence of autoantibodies against acetylcholine (ACh) receptors at the neuromuscular junction (NMJ). The most common finding in myasthenia gravis is fatigability (i.e. muscles become gradually weaker with activity). Extraocular and facial muscles are commonly involved. Ptosis, diplopia, dysarthria and dysphagia can occur, with death usually occurring because of respiratory muscle failure. Acetylcholinesterase inhibitors (e.g. neostigmine and physostigmine) can be used in the management of myasthenia gravis. They work by preventing the breakdown of ACh in the synaptic cleft, increasing its availability for transmission at the NMJ.

48. C – Dissociation of ribosomes
Dissociation of ribosomes from the endoplasmic reticulum is characteristic of reversible cell injury. Irreversible cell injury leads to one of two endpoints, apoptosis or necrosis. Apoptosis is programmed cell death and is orderly in nature in comparison to necrosis, which is a traumatic form of cell death secondary to pathological stimuli, such as hypoxia, and is random and diffuse in nature.

49. B – BRCA1
The BRCA1 (Breast Cancer 1, early onset) tumour suppressor gene has been implicated in breast and ovarian cancer. It is inherited as an autosomal dominant gene and is located on chromosome 17q. Carriers of BRCA1 have a lifetime risk approaching 80% of developing breast cancer and a 40–60% increased risk of developing ovarian cancer.

50. A – Amitriptyline
Amitriptyline is a tricyclic antidepressant used in the management of chronic neuralgia. Side-effects are predominantly antimuscarinic and cardiovascular. An example of its use with regard to neuropathic pain management is for those who suffer with chronic functional abdominal pain. An alternative agent of choice is gabapentin.

Questions Paper 2

1. Which of the following is true of lipopeptide antibiotics?
   A. They are effective against Gram-negative bacteria.
   B. They are effective against Gram-positive bacteria.
   C. They are primarily excreted by the liver.
   D. They are unable to bind protein.
   E. They are unable to bind to the cell membrane.

2. Which type of ion channels do local anaesthetic agents target?
   A. Calcium channels
   B. Gamma-aminobutyric acid gated chloride channels
   C. N-Methyl-D-aspartate cation channels
   D. Potassium channels
   E. Sodium channels

3. Which one of the following drugs is a specific inhibitor of bacterial dihydrofolate reductase?
   A. Methotrexate
   B. Nitisinone
   C. Pemetrexed
   D. Proguanil
   E. Trimethoprim

4. Metastatic spread of cancer via the blood to the bone can be caused by which of the following tumours most commonly?
   A. Brain
   B. Lung
   C. Neurofibroma
   D. Oesophagus
   E. Thyroid

5. Which one of the following functions do osteoblasts perform?
   A. Exchange of nutrients and waste products
   B. Production of osteoid
   C. Release of hydrogen ions
   D. Resorption of bone
   E. Secretion of cathepsin K

6. Quinolones inhibit which part of nucleic acid synthesis?
    A. They inhibit dihydrofolate reductase.
    B. They inhibit dihydropteroate synthetase.
    C. They inhibit DNA gyrase.
    D. They inhibit DNA synthesis by reducing a nitro group and forming reactive intermediates.
    E. They inhibit RNA polymerase.

7. Which of the following statements regarding blood supply to the brain is *incorrect*?
    A. The internal carotid artery arises from the common carotid artery at the level of the suprasternal notch.
    B. The ophthalmic artery is a branch of the internal carotid artery.
    C. The middle cerebral arteries supply the lateral cortex.
    D. The posterior cerebral arteries supply the visual cortex.
    E. The vertebral arteries are branches of the subclavian artery.

8. Which vessel begins beyond the inguinal ligament, and then runs in the adductor canal before changing its name as it passes through the hiatus in adductor magnus?
    A. Anterior tibial artery
    B. Femoral artery
    C. Popliteal artery
    D. Posterior tibial artery
    E. Profundus femoris

9. Which one of the following statements regarding skeletal muscle structure is correct?
    A. Actin filaments are thicker than myosin filaments.
    B. Sarcomeres are made up of many myofibrils.
    C. The sarcomere is made up of light and dark bands; the light parts consist of actin filaments.
    D. Thick filaments are composed of four heavy chains of myosin and a regulatory light chain.
    E. Z lines anchor the thick myosin filaments.

10. Which one of the following muscles facilitates flexion of the hip joint and extension at the knee?
    A. The biceps femoris
    B. The rectus femoris
    C. The sartorius
    D. The semimembranosus
    E. The semitendinosus

11. In which phase of the cell cycle is DNA synthesized?
    A. G_0 phase
    B. G_1 phase

C. G_2 phase
D. S phase
E. None of the above

12. Which artery has multiple branches partly or wholly supplying a number of structures including the face, tongue and thyroid?
   A. Common carotid
   B. External carotid
   C. Internal carotid
   D. Subclavian artery
   E. Vertebral artery

13. Which one of the following statements regarding the musculature of the lower limb is correct?
   A. Contraction of the psoas major results in extension of the hip.
   B. The femoral nerve supplies the hamstring muscles.
   C. The iliacus, the adductor longus and the inguinal ligament border the femoral triangle.
   D. The sartorius facilitates sitting cross-legged.
   E. The sciatic nerve supplies the quadriceps muscles.

14. Muscles are composed of fast and slow muscle fibres. Which one of the following statements regarding fast and slow fibres is correct?
   A. Fast fibres are red in colour because of large amounts of myoglobin.
   B. Fast fibres are smaller for quicker release of energy.
   C. Slow fibres are adapted for prolonged muscle contraction.
   D. Slow fibres have fewer mitochondria than fast fibres.
   E. Slow fibres undergo only anaerobic metabolism.

15. I-bands consist of:
   A. Actin
   B. Actin and myosin
   C. Myosin
   D. Myosin and tropomyosin
   E. Myosin and troponin

16. Which of the following is responsible for producing adenosine triphosphate?
   A. Golgi apparatus
   B. Mitochondria
   C. Nucleus
   D. Ribosome
   E. Rough endoplasmic reticulum

17. Acetylcholine is an agonist for which target receptor?
   A. $5HT_2$ receptor
   B. Beta adrenoceptor

C. Histamine receptor
D. Nicotinic receptor
E. μ-Receptor

18. Which enzyme is the drug target for statins?
    A. Choline acetyltransferase
    B. Cyclooxygenase
    C. DOPA decarboxylase
    D. HMG-CoA reductase
    E. Xanthine oxidase

19. The primary function of which of the following is the processing and packaging of macromolecules?
    A. Golgi apparatus
    B. Mitochondria
    C. Nucleus
    D. Rough endoplasmic reticulum
    E. Smooth endoplasmic reticulum

20. In respiratory alkalosis which ion is decreased in concentration?
    A. Calcium
    B. Magnesium
    C. Phosphate
    D. Potassium
    E. Sodium

21. Which of the following statements about myelinated axons is true?
    A. Action potential conduction is slower
    B. Axon diameter is smaller
    C. More adenosine triphosphate is needed for repolarization
    D. More energy is needed for depolarization of the membrane
    E. They are contained only within the central nervous system

22. A sarcomere is defined as the interval between two adjacent:
    A. A-bands
    B. I-bands
    C. Thick filaments
    D. Thin filaments
    E. Z-lines

23. Which of the following can occur with the use of the tumour necrosis factor-α inhibitor infliximab?
    A. Chronic autoimmune disease
    B. Diabetes insipidus
    C. Infertility
    D. Reactivation of tuberculosis
    E. Rhabdomyolysis

24. Which one of the following drugs does *not* inhibit dihydrofolate reductase?
   A. Allopurinol
   B. Methotrexate
   C. Pemetrexed
   D. Proguanil
   E. Trimethoprim

25. The *APC* tumour suppressor gene is located on which chromosome?
   A. 17p
   B. 5q
   C. 7q
   D. 13q
   E. 17q

26. Which one of the following complement pathways would activate C3 via bacterial lipopolysaccharides?
   A. Alternative pathway
   B. Apoptosis
   C. Classical pathway
   D. Lectin pathway
   E. Tyrosine kinase pathway

27. Which of the following is true with regard to local potentials?
   A. Summation of local potentials results in inhibition of an impulse.
   B. The strength of electrical potential is lowest at the point of initiation.
   C. The strength of initiating stimulus has no effect on the magnitude of the potential.
   D. The strength of the potential increases with increasing distance from the site of initiation.
   E. They can travel in both directions along an axon.

28. Which of the following describes the resting potential within a neuron?
   A. −30 mV
   B. −55 mV
   C. −70 mV
   D. −90 mV
   E. +50 mV

29. Which of the following is true of β-lactam antibiotics?
   A. The cell wall is unaffected by their action.
   B. They are effective against mycobacteria.
   C. They are effective against slow dividing bacteria.
   D. They are not thought to be bactericidal.
   E. They inhibit the enzymes which are involved in the third stage of cell wall synthesis.

30. Which of the following is an atypical antipsychotic drug?
    A. Chlorpromazine
    B. Flupentixol
    C. Fluphenazine
    D. Haloperidol
    E. Olanzapine

31. The *p53* tumour suppressor gene is located on which chromosome?
    A. 17p
    B. 5q
    C. 7q
    D. 13q
    E. 17q

32. When an action potential reaches a synapse, what is directly responsible for triggering the exocytosis of neurosecretory vesicles into the synaptic cleft?
    A. G-protein signal transduction
    B. Increased Ca^{2+} within the presynaptic cytoplasm
    C. Increased Na^+ within the presynaptic cleft
    D. Increased production of acetylcholine
    E. The influence of noradrenaline

33. Which one of the following is *not* a function of mitochondria?
    A. Calcium signalling
    B. Cellular differentiation
    C. Cellular migration
    D. Production of adenosine triphosphate
    E. Programmed cell death

34. Which one of the following is *not* an end product of arachidonic acid metabolism?
    A. Laminin
    B. Leukotriene
    C. Prostacyclin
    D. Prostaglandin
    E. Thromboxane

35. Which structure is *not* found in the broad ligament?
    A. Ovarian ligament
    B. Ovary
    C. Uterine artery
    D. Uterine tube
    E. Uterovaginal nerve plexus

36. Which of the following is *not* a branch of the internal carotid artery?
    A. Anterior cerebral artery
    B. Anterior choroidal artery
    C. Middle cerebral artery

D. Posterior cerebral artery

E. Posterior communicating artery

37. The vertebral arteries unite at the lower border of the pons to give rise to which one of the following?

A. Anterior spinal artery

B. Basilar artery

C. Cerebellar artery

D. Posterior cerebral artery

E. Posterior spinal artery

38. Which of the following gives the correct sequence of mitosis?

A. Prophase, anaphase, metaphase, telophase

B. Prophase, anaphase, telophase, metaphase

C. Prophase, metaphase, anaphase, telophase

D. Telophase, anaphase, prophase, metaphase

E. Telophase, prophase, anaphase, metaphase

39. Which of the following is the chief inhibitory neurotransmitter in the central nervous system?

A. Acetylcholine

B. Dopamine

C. Gamma-aminobutyric acid

D. Serotonin

E. Zinc

40. Which one of the following is *not* an effect mediated by activation of the complement cascade?

A. Activation and chemotaxis of leukocytes

B. Alteration of the hypothalamic thermostat

C. Cell lysis of microbes

D. Increased vascular permeability

E. Phagocytosis

41. Which one of the following is the most common outcome of acute inflammation?

A. Abscess formation

B. Organization

C. Progression to chronic inflammation

D. Resolution

E. Suppuration

42. Which enzyme is the drug target for aspirin?

A. Acetylcholinesterase

B. Angiotensin-converting enzyme

C. Cyclooxygenase

D. Monoamine oxidase

E. Thymidine kinase

43. Which one of the following target receptors is intracellular?
    A. Gamma-aminobutyric acid A receptor
    B. Insulin receptor
    C. Muscarinic acetylcholine receptor
    D. Nicotinic acetylcholine receptor
    E. Steroid receptor

44. Which statement best describes the ovaries?
    A. The left ovarian vein joins the inferior vena cava.
    B. The ovarian artery anastomoses with the internal iliac artery.
    C. They are lined by peritoneum.
    D. They are supplied by the ovarian artery, a branch of the abdominal aorta.
    E. They lie within the broad ligament.

45. Which one of the following statements concerning the uterus is *false*?
    A. It is connected to the vagina via the cervix.
    B. It is normally retroverted.
    C. It is primarily supplied by the uterine artery.
    D. It is supported by the urogenital and pelvic diaphragm.
    E. The anterior surface is related to the bladder.

46. Which medium vessel vasculitis gives rise to microaneurysms and fibroid necrosis of vessels walls, is associated with hepatitis B antigenaemia and primarily affects middle-aged men?
    A. Classical polyarteritis nodosum
    B. Giant cell arteritis
    C. Kawasaki disease
    D. Takayasu arteritis
    E. Wegener granulomatosis

47. The synthesis of prostaglandins and thromboxanes is stimulated by which enzyme?
    A. Cyclooxygenase
    B. HMG-CoA reductase
    C. Lipoxygenase
    D. Myeloperoxidase
    E. Xanthine oxidase

48. Deficiency in complement C3 would make a patient more susceptible to which one of the following?
    A. Bacterial infection
    B. Parasitic infection
    C. Prion disease
    D. Systemic lupus erythematosus
    E. Virus infection

49. What term is most commonly applied to the vascular aneurysms that may be seen in syphilis infection?
   A. Berry
   B. Connective tissue abnormality
   C. Cystic medial degeneration
   D. False
   E. Mycotic

50. Which of the following conditions is associated with granulomatous inflammation of the aorta and its major branches?
   A. Classical polyarteritis nodosum
   B. Giant cell arteritis
   C. Kawasaki disease
   D. Takayasu arteritis
   E. Wegener granulomatosis

Answers Paper 2

1. B – They are effective against Gram-positive bacteria
Daptomycin is an example of a novel lipopeptide antibiotic. The activity of these agents is limited to Gram-positive bacteria. Lipopeptide antibiotics bind to the cell membrane, creating disruptions that allow ion leakage. This results in rapid depolarization with a consequent loss of the membrane potential which inhibits protein, RNA and DNA synthesis.

2. E – Sodium channels
Local anaesthetic agents, such as lidocaine, block voltage-gated sodium channels to prevent the depolarization required for action potential generation. As a result, neurotransmission is blocked.

3. E – Trimethoprim
Tetrahydrofolic acid is an essential precursor for the synthesis of DNA, and dihydrofolate reductase is an enzyme in the metabolic pathway that produces tetrahydrofolic acid. Inhibiting dihydrofolate reductase stops the synthesis of this folic acid, thus depleting the precursors available for DNA synthesis. Trimethoprim specifically acts on bacterial dihydrofolate reductase, thus depleting bacteria of folic acid. As bacteria are unable to use folic acid from the host, they are unable to synthesize DNA and repli cate. As such, trimethoprim is a bacteriostatic antimicrobial.

4. E – Thyroid
Tumours that spread to the bony skeleton via the bloodstream usually arise from the bronchus, breast, thyroid, kidney or prostate. Bony metastases are problematic as they can result in severe intractable pain, bony fractures, hypercalcaemia and cord compression. It is difficult for cancer cells to survive outside their region of origin, so in order to metastasize they must find a location with similar characteristics. For example, breast tumours which gathered calcium ions from breast milk can metastasize to bones and gather calcium from the bone.

5. B – Production of osteoid
Osteoblasts are the cells responsible for bone formation. They do this by producing osteoid (mainly type I collagen). They arise from progenitor cells within the bone marrow and periosteum. As they become mature cells they express different proteins, such as osteopontin and osteocalcin, which are involved in various phases of bone regulation. Osteoblasts become osteocytes when they become part of the matrix into which they secrete.

They are able to degrade bone though a rapid mechanism called osteocytic osteolysis. Osteoclasts are responsible for the removal of bone tissue. This occurs through the resorption of organic bone. They also secrete cathepsin K which is involved in the lysis of collagen. Through the action of carbonic anhydrase, osteoclasts release hydrogen ions. This allows the dissolution of the bone matrix.

6. C – They inhibit DNA gyrase

Quinolones inhibit DNA gyrase (also known as DNA topoisomerase II, an enzyme required in DNA unwinding). Trimethoprim and methotrexate inhibit dihydrofolate reductase. Sulphonamides inhibit dihydropteroate synthetase. Rifampicin inhibits RNA polymerase. 5-Nitroimidazoles (such as metronidazole) inhibit DNA synthesis by reducing a nitro group and forming reactive intermediates.

7. A – The internal carotid artery arises from the common carotid artery at the level of the suprasternal notch

The internal carotid artery is a branch of the common carotid artery, but arises at the level of the third cervical vertebra. The suprasternal notch is at the T2/3 vertebral level. The internal carotid arteries can be divided into seven segments according to the Bouthillier classification. The seven parts comprise the following (from proximal to distal): cervical segment; petrous segment; lacerum segment; cavernous segment; clinoid segment; ophthalmic (supraclinoid) segment; and the communicating (terminal) segment.

8. B – Femoral artery

The femoral artery is the continuation of the external iliac artery below the inguinal ligament. It passes through the femoral canal, accompanied by the femoral vein, femoral nerve and lymphatics. The anatomy of this area is of everyday clinical relevance, particularly with reference to acupuncture, arteriopuncture, central line insertion and hernia formation. A useful mnemonic for the order of the structures within the femoral canal is 'NAVY' (nerve, artery, vein, Y-fronts – running lateral to medial). The femoral artery initially runs anteriorly before passing under sartorius to the gap in adductor magnus and entering the popliteal fossa – this passage beneath sartorius and through adductor magnus is the adductor (or Hunter's) canal.

9. C – The sarcomere is made up of light and dark bands; the light parts consisting of actin filaments

Skeletal muscle is striated and made up of myofibrils, which are divided into sarcomeres. Each sarcomere is divided from the next by the Z line, composed of actinins, which anchors the thin filaments. ('Z' is from the German *Zwischenscheibe* = the disc in between.) Thin filaments are made of actin, while the thick comprise mainly myosin. Thick and thin filaments are arranged so that they interdigitate with one another.

Light bands are made up of thin filaments, while the dark bands comprise overlapping myosin and actin. Muscle contraction is brought about by thin filaments moving over the thick filaments via ATP-dependent cross-bridge formation.

10. B – The rectus femoris
The rectus femoris muscle is innervated by the femoral nerve and allows flexion at the hip joint. Its insertion into the quadriceps tendon also facilitates knee extension. Rectus femoris is one of the four components of the quadriceps femoris, the other three being vastus lateralis, vastus medialis and vastus intermedius. The semimembranosus, the semitendinosus and the biceps femoris make up the hamstring muscles, which facilitate knee flexion and hip extension.

11. D – S phase
DNA replication occurs during the S (synthesis) phase of the cell cycle. During this phase, there is also initiation of protein synthesis and replication of organelles.

12. B   External carotid
The common carotid bifurcates into the internal and external carotid arteries above the level of the thyroid cartilage. The external carotid has multiple branches providing vascular supply to the throat, mouth and external structures of the head.

13. D   The sartorius facilitates sitting cross-legged
The sartorius muscle, etymologically the 'tailor's muscle', enables hip flexion and lateral rotation, as well as flexion at the knee. It is innervated by the femoral nerve, attaches to the anterior superior iliac spine and runs inferomedially. The femoral triangle contains the femoral nerve, artery and vein, in addition to the deep inguinal lymph nodes. It is bordered by the inguinal ligament anteriorly, the adductor longus medially and the sartorius laterally. The quadriceps are supplied by the femoral nerve and cause knee extension, while knee flexion and hip extension are controlled by the hamstrings, which are supplied by the sciatic nerve.

14. C – Slow fibres are adapted for prolonged muscle contraction
Slow fibres are also known as red muscle because of their high levels of myoglobin. They have a large number of mitochondria for high levels of oxidative metabolism. Fast fibres, or white muscle, are larger and have large amounts of glycolytic enzymes for the rapid release of energy. Fast fibres are used for short-acting, powerful muscle contractions.

15. A – Actin
Thick myofilaments lie between the thin myofilaments. The partial interdigitation between the thin and thick myofilaments gives the appearance of the light and dark bands which give striated skeletal muscle its name (Latin *striae* = furrows). Light I-bands are portions of actin which do not

overlap with myosin. Dark A-bands, on the other hand, represent the filaments of actin which overlap with the myosin filaments. The 'I' and 'A' stand for *isotropic* and *anisotropic* – terms which relate to their properties under polarized microscopy.

16. B – Mitochondria

Mitochondria are responsible for the production of adenosine triphosphate (ATP), which is a cell's source of energy. The nucleus contains most of a cell's genetic material and is a membrane-enclosed organelle. A ribosome is responsible for the production of proteins from amino acids. They are divided into two subunits. The smaller of the two binds to messenger RNA and the larger binds to transfer RNA. Rough endoplasmic reticulum is so called because of the presence of ribosomes bound to its surface. They are not a stable part of the structure as they are constantly being released from the membrane.

17. D – Nicotinic receptor

Acetylcholine is an agonist for nicotinic receptors. Nicotinic receptors are thus part of the class of cholinergic receptors, with muscarinic receptors being the other predominant member. Nicotinic receptors are commonly found at neuromuscular junctions, and activation by acetylcholine leads to an influx of sodium and a resultant action potential.

18. D – HMG-CoA reductase

HMG-CoA (3-hydroxy-3-methylglutaryl-coenzyme A) reductase is an enzyme involved in the biosynthesis of cholesterol. Statins are competitive inhibitors of this enzyme, thus the drug reduces cholesterol synthesis and is widely used in treating hypercholesterolaemia. Statins not only lower cholesterol by directly reducing synthesis through competitive inhibition of the enzyme, but also by increasing uptake of low-density lipoproteins (LDLs). This is because the reduced synthesis of cholesterol means the body upregulates LDL receptors, which has the beneficial effect of increasing LDL uptake from the blood.

19. A – Golgi apparatus

The Golgi apparatus processes and packages macromolecules, such as proteins, for their subsequent secretion or use within the cell. Mitochondria are responsible for the production of ATP which is the cell's source of energy. The nucleus contains most of a cell's genetic material and is a membrane-enclosed organelle. A ribosome is responsible for the production of proteins from amino acids. Rough endoplasmic reticulum is so called because of the presence of ribosomes bound to its surface.

20. A – Calcium

As the pH rises through the elimination of carbon dioxide, there is a concomitant decrease in the ionized calcium concentration. In alkalosis, the protein in the blood becomes ionized into anions. This causes free calcium present in blood to bind strongly to protein, leading to tetany if severe.

21. B – Axon diameter is smaller

Myelinated neurons are found both within the central nervous system (CNS) and peripheral nervous system (PNS). They allow faster action potential conduction and consume lower levels of energy and ATP. This is because only a small portion of membrane needs to undergo depolarization and repolarization, as the action potential can jump between areas of myelin insulation ('saltatory conduction'). Because action potential conduction is faster in myelinated neurons, their diameter can be smaller without compromising speed. This allows greater space efficiency.

22. E – Z-lines

Skeletal muscle fibres consist of several smaller subunits called myofibrils. These myofibrils are a series of parallel subunits that contain the contractile proteins of the skeletal muscle fibre. When viewed closely, myofibrils have a striated appearance with light and dark bands. The light bands are called I-bands and consist of thin myofilaments composed predominantly of actin, with troponin and tropomyosin. The dark bands are called A-bands and are made up of thick myofilaments which consist mainly of myosin. The Z-line is a line which dissects each I-band. The interval between two adjacent Z-lines is called a sarcomere, and this is the basic contractile unit of skeletal muscle.

23. D – Reactivation of tuberculosis

Infliximab is a cytokine modulator that inhibits tumour necrosis factor-α (TNF-α) and is used in the management of rheumatoid arthritis and Crohn disease. Because it dampens the immune response, it predisposes to infection. It has been shown to reactivate latent tuberculosis so patients must be assessed for the presence of infection before commencing infliximab. Reactivation of latent TB is highest in the first twelve months of treatment. All patients commenced on anti-TNF therapies need to be closely monitored for TB. This needs to continue for 6 months after discontinuing infliximab treatment due to the prolonged elimination phase of infliximab.

24. A – Allopurinol

Dihydrofolate reductase is an enzyme used in the synthetic pathway of purines, required for DNA synthesis. Trimethoprim acts on bacterial dihydrofolate reductase, methotrexate and pemetrexed work on human dihydrofolate reductase, while proguanil works on parasitic dihydrofolate reductase. As a result of this specificity, each has different clinical indications, e.g. trimethoprim is used to treat bacterial infections, whereas proguanil is used to treat parasitic infections like malaria. Allopurinol is a xanthine oxidase inhibitor and is used to treat gout.

25. B – 5q

The tumour suppressor gene named *APC* (adenomatous polyposis coli) is located on chromosome 5q. It is inherited in an autosomal dominant fashion and results in the formation of hundreds to thousands of tubular adenomas within the colon. These adenomatous polyps are 100% premalignant and need to be surgically excised to prevent progression to cancer.

26. A – Alternative pathway
Complement C3 is cleaved to form C3a and C3b within plasma. The alternative complement pathway is triggered by C3b binding. C3b can attach to cell surfaces, but is inhibited by sialic acid on mammalian cell surfaces. Some microbes and virus cell membranes lack sialic acid. To this end, C3b can bind lipopolysaccharide on Gram-negative bacteria and independently initiate the complement cascade more quickly than via antibody activation.

27. E – They can travel in both directions along an axon
Before electrical signals are formed, there has to be a change in cell charge from the resting membrane potential. Local potentials are generated by chemical, mechanical or electrical inputs received by the neuron causing small depolarizations. The electrical currents produced can travel in either direction along an axon. The strength of the potential generated depends upon the strength of the input, and as a result they are maximally strong at the point of generation. The strength of the potential quickly diminishes the further the signal travels from its original source. Summation of local potentials, rather than inhibiting an impulse, is a way to increase their strength.

28. C – –70 mV
The resting potential of a neuron membrane is –70 mV, close to the equilibrium potential for potassium ions (–90 mV, dictated by the Nernst equation). In order for an action potential to be generated, the threshold level of –55 mV within a neuron has to be reached. Myocytes have a resting potential of –90 mV. The equilibrium potential for sodium is +70 mV. As the membrane depolarizes and more Na^+ ions enter the neuron, its membrane potential will become closer to this level.

29. C – They are effective against slow dividing bacteria
Bacterial cell walls are made from peptidoglycans. These peptidoglycans are essential for cell wall structural integrity, and the consequent inhibition of synthesis by β-lactam antibiotics leads to bacterial death.

30. E – Olanzapine
Atypical antipsychotics are so called because they work differently from typical antipsychotics, but most affect serotonin and dopamine receptors.

31. A – 17p
The *p53* (protein 53) tumour suppressor gene, which is implicated in more than 50% of all cancers, is located on chromosome 17 (17p13.1). The *p53* gene is also known as the guardian of the genome because it has such an important role in cell regulation. The *p53* gene is responsible for activating DNA repair proteins – it can arrest cell growth by stopping the cell

cycle at the G_1/S phase, allowing damaged DNA to be repaired. The *p53* gene is also responsible for activating apoptosis in response to severely damaged DNA.

32. B – Increased Ca^{2+} within the presynaptic cytoplasm

Depolarization of the presynaptic membrane via an influx of Na^+ results in the opening of voltage-gated Ca^{2+} channels. Increased Ca^{2+} within the cytoplasm encourages exocytosis.

33. C – Cellular migration

Mitochondria have a central role in the production of ATP. They are also vitally important in the regulation of the membrane potential, apoptosis, calcium signalling, cellular proliferation and steroid synthesis. They are not, however, involved in cellular migration.

34. A – Laminin

Laminins are glycoproteins essential for the structure of the basal lamina (part of the basement membrane). They are coded for, and produced by, various cells involved within the inflammatory response.

35. B – Ovary

The ovaries are not part of the broad ligament, but are attached to the broad ligament via a fold of the peritoneum known as the mesovarium.

36. D – Posterior cerebral artery

The posterior cerebral artery is a terminal branch of the basilar artery. All the other arteries are branches of the internal carotid artery.

37. B – Basilar artery

The basilar artery is formed through the unification of the two vertebral arteries at the base of the lower border of the pons. It gives rise to several branches including the anterior inferior cerebellar, superior cerebellar, labyrinthine and the posterior cerebral arteries.

38. C – Prophase, metaphase, anaphase, telophase

The correct sequence of mitosis is prophase, metaphase, anaphase and telophase. The key features of each are as follows:

- Prophase: chromatin condensation and mitotic spindle formation
- Metaphase: chromosome alignment at the equator of the spindle
- Anaphase: sister chromatids are separated and migrate to opposite poles
- Telophase: sister chromatids arrive at the spindles and decondense

39. C – Gamma-aminobutyric acid

Gamma-aminobutyric acid (GABA) is the required neurotransmitter at the majority of fast inhibitory synapses of the central nervous system. Serotonin, dopamine and acetylcholine are the excitatory neurotransmitters in the nervous system. Zinc is not a neurotransmitter.

40. B – Alteration of the hypothalamic thermostat
Alteration of the hypothalamic thermostat is produced by several cytokines including interleukin 2 (IL-2) and tumour necrosis factor alpha (TNF-α) but is not a consequence of complement activation.

41. D – Resolution
Resolution occurs following minimal tissue damage and results in complete tissue regeneration to its original function and structure. This is the most common outcome. Suppuration and abscess formation occur when an infective agent persists within a tissue. Organization describes the process by which the components of a tissue are replaced with fibrous or scar tissue. Progression to chronic inflammation occurs if the causative agent is not able to be removed.

42. C – Cyclooxygenase
Aspirin is an inhibitor of cyclooxygenase (COX). Aspirin irreversibly acetylates part of the active site of COX-1 and changes the activity of COX-2, rendering the enzyme incapable of further successful enzyme–substrate reactions. COX is an enzyme involved in the production of prostaglandins and thromboxanes. Aspirin is thus able to reduce the production of these, resulting in an anti-inflammatory, antipyretic, anti-inflammatory and antiplatelet activity.

43. E – Steroid receptor
All the options listed, apart from steroid receptors, are membrane receptors. The steroid receptors are all intracellular nuclear receptors and influence gene transcription. Intracellular steroid receptors comprise a DNA binding domain, variable domain, hinge region and hormone binding domain. The hinge region is known to control receptor movement, whereas the DNA binding domain controls gene activation. The domain comprises zinc and cysteine residues.

44. D – They are supplied by the ovarian artery, a branch of the abdominal aorta
The ovaries are not lined by peritoneum, and thus an oocyte is released into the peritoneal cavity. The anterior surface of the ovary is attached to the broad ligament via a fold of the peritoneum (the mesovarium). The left ovarian vein drains into the left renal vein, while the right ovarian vein directly joins the inferior vena cava (a similar distribution pattern to the testicular veins). The ovarian artery anastomoses with the uterine artery.

45. B – It is normally retroverted
The uterus is normally anteverted and anteflexed. It is only retroverted in around 20% of women. All the other given statements are true.

46. A – Classical polyarteritis nodosum
Polyarteritis nodosa is a medium vessel vasculitis. It is most common in adult males and is often seen in association with hepatitis B infection.

Immune complex deposition causes a type III hypersensitivity reaction. There can be systemic involvement, but a classic exam presentation is a middle-aged man presenting with abdominal pain and renal failure.

47. A – Cyclooxygenase

Cyclooxygenase (COX) is the enzyme required to synthesise prostaglandins and thromboxanes. Xanthine oxidase catalyses the oxidation of xanthine to uric acid. Allopurinol, used in the prevention of gout, is a xanthine oxidase inhibitor. HMG-CoA reductase converts HMG-CoA to mevalonic acid, and this is an important step in cholesterol formation. Statins are HMG-CoA reductase inhibitors. Myeloperoxidase (MPO) is contained in neutrophils and produces hypochlorous acid from hydrogen peroxide to enable the oxidative killing of microbes. Lipoxygenase enables the production of leukotrienes from arachidonic acid.

48. A – Bacterial infection

Reduction in complement C3 results in a reduced ability to eliminate microbes via opsonization and the membrane attack complex. This is a large component of the body's immune response to bacterial invasion. Effective deficiency of C3 can also occur with a deficiency of factor H or factor I (inhibitors of complement activation) due to the inappropriate activation of C3 via the alternative pathway. Deficiency of C1 predisposes an individual to SLE, because there is less opsonization of immune complexes via the classical pathway. This reduces the number of soluble immune complexes, encouraging their precipitation within tissues.

49. E – Mycotic

Initially, *mycotic* was a term reserved for fungal aneurysms but it is now commonly applied to all aneurysms with infective aetiology. Later stages of syphilis infection can lead to loss of the vasa vasorum within the aorta and other large arteries, leading to aneurysms of these vessels.

50. D – Takayasu arteritis

Takayasu arteritis, often known as pulseless disease or aortic arch syndrome, is classified as a large vessel vasculitis. It chiefly affects females, the classic presentation being in young Asian women. The aetiology is unknown and the disease is rare. It causes granulomatous inflammation of the aorta and its major branches, giving rise to difficulty in palpation of some of the peripheral pulses.

Questions Paper 3

1. Which of the following drugs is a chimeric monoclonal antibody directed against platelets?
   A. Abciximab
   B. Aspirin
   C. Dipyridamole
   D. Indomethacin
   E. Prasugrel

2. From which area of the oral cavity does the glossopharyngeal nerve convey the sensation of taste?
   A. The anterior two-thirds of the tongue
   B. The back of the oral cavity
   C. The lateral sides of the tongue
   D. The posterior one-third of the tongue
   E. The posterior two-thirds of the tongue

3. Which of the following movements is facilitated by teres major?
   A. Abductor of the shoulder joint
   B. Extension at the elbow joint
   C. Flexor of the shoulder joint
   D. Lateral rotation of the shoulder
   E. Medial rotation of the shoulder

4. Which pulse is found midway between the anterior superior iliac spine and the pubic symphysis?
   A. Brachial
   B. Carotid
   C. Femoral
   D. Popliteal
   E. Radial

5. Which of the following is the area between two adjoining cells which forms an impermeable barrier to fluid?
   A. Desmosomes
   B. Gap junction
   C. Zonula adherens
   D. Zonula occludens
   E. None of the above

6. Which one of the following collagen types is present in hyaline cartilage?
   A. Type I collagen
   B. Type II collagen
   C. Type III collagen
   D. Type IV collagen
   E. Type V collagen

7. Which one of the following is a non-immune function of the lymphatic system?
   A. Electrolyte balance
   B. Fat transport
   C. Glucose homeostasis
   D. Protein absorption
   E. Toxin degradation

8. To which one of the following drugs used in the treatment of heart failure do people often develop tolerance?
   A. Carvedilol
   B. Enalapril
   C. Furosemide
   D. Isosorbide mononitrate
   E. Metoprolol

9. Which of the following electrolyte abnormalities can increase the likelihood of digoxin toxicity?
   A. Hypercalcaemia
   B. Hyperkalaemia
   C. Hypermagnesemia
   D. Hypocalcaemia
   E. Hyponatraemia

10. Which is the most common type of laryngeal carcinoma?
    A. Adenocarcinoma
    B. Basal cell carcinoma
    C. Squamous cell carcinoma
    D. Verrucous carcinoma
    E. None of the above

11. Which one of the following is present within a keratinocyte?
    A. Basal lamina
    B. Costamere
    C. Desmosome
    D. Hemidesmosome
    E. None of the above

12. Which one of the following is an immigrant cell of connective tissue?
    A. Adipocyte
    B. Fibroblast

C. Macrophage
D. Mast cell
E. Monocyte

13. At which vertebral level does the trachea commence?
    A. C5
    B. C6
    C. C7
    D. C8
    E. T1

14. Tardive dyskinesia is *least* associated with which of the following drugs?
    A. Clozapine
    B. Haloperidol
    C. Olanzapine
    D. Quetiapine
    E. Risperidone

15. In a patient with depression at a high risk of taking an overdose, which one of the following antidepressant classes would be the safest to prescribe?
    A. Benzodiazepines
    B. Monoamine oxidase inhibitors
    C. Selective serotonin reuptake inhibitors
    D. Serotonin–noradrenaline reuptake inhibitors
    E. Tricyclic antidepressants

16. A female patient has been started on a new medication by her GP. She returns 3 weeks later stating that since she has started on this drug she has muscle pain and wishes to stop taking the drug. Which drug has she most likely been started on?
    A. Digoxin
    B. Metoprolol
    C. Ramipril
    D. Simvastatin
    E. Spironolactone

17. A male patient is well controlled on warfarin for his atrial fibrillation. Which of the following drugs is known to increasing the INR in patients taking warfarin?
    A. Allopurinol
    B. Carbamazepine
    C. Phenobarbital
    D. Phenytoin
    E. Rifampicin

18. Which of the following is *not* a branch vessel associated directly or indirectly with the internal iliac artery?
    A. Inferior rectal artery
    B. Inferior vesical artery
    C. Internal pudendal artery
    D. Superior vesical artery
    E. Testicular artery

19. Which of the following are found at the base of the intestinal crypts and contain large acidophilic granules?
    A. Enterocytes
    B. Enteroendocrine cells
    C. Goblet cells
    D. Paneth cells
    E. Stem cells

20. Which one of the following contains cadherins which encircle the cell?
    A. Desmosomes
    B. Gap junction
    C. Tight junctions
    D. Zonula adherens
    E. None of the above

21. Which of the following statements regarding heart valves is correct?
    A. The aortic and mitral valves both have three leaflets.
    B. The aortic and pulmonary valves are tricuspid.
    C. The aortic, mitral and tricuspid valves all have three leaflets.
    D. The aortic valve is the only cardiac valve to have three leaflets.
    E. The pulmonary and mitral valves are bicuspid.

22. Which of the following muscles is *not* supplied by the median nerve?
    A. The abductor pollicis brevis
    B. The adductor pollicis brevis
    C. The flexor pollicis brevis
    D. The opponens pollicis
    E. The pronator teres

23. Use of which one of the following drugs is an absolute contraindication in bilateral renal artery stenosis?
    A. Amlodipine
    B. Bendroflumethiazide
    C. Bisoprolol
    D. Carvedilol
    E. Ramipril

24. Which one of the following statements regarding analgesia is correct?
    A. Fentanyl is a synthetic opioid commonly used in anaesthesia.
    B. Morphine is a first-line agent in the treatment of headaches.

C. Paracetamol is effective in treating severe pain.

D. Peptic ulceration is a common side-effect of fentanyl use.

E. Respiratory depression is a common consequence of non-steroidal anti-inflammatory drug use.

25. Horner's syndrome results in a triad of signs due to loss of the sympathetic innervation. These are:

A. Pupillary constriction, drooping of eyelid and loss of sweating around affected eye

B. Pupillary constriction, retraction of eyelid and loss of sweating around both eyes

C. Pupillary relaxation, drooping of eyelid and loss of sweating around affected eye

D. Pupillary relaxation, retraction of eyelid and loss of sweating around both eyes

E. None of the above

26. From which area of the tongue does the facial nerve convey the sensation of taste?

A. The anterior two-thirds of the tongue

B. The centre of the tongue

C. The lateral sides of the tongue

D. The posterior one-third of the tongue

E. The posterior two-thirds of the tongue

27. Which one of the following nerves supplies the gluteus maximus?

A. The femoral nerve

B. The inferior gluteal nerve

C. The obturator nerve

D. The sciatic nerve

E. The superior gluteal nerve

28. Which of the following best describes the location of the atrioventricular node?

A. Positioned between the atria and ventricles in the posteroinferior region of the interatrial septum, near the opening of the coronary sinus

B. Positioned between the atria and ventricles in the ventricular septum

C. Positioned in the inferior wall of the right atrium lateral to the tricuspid valve

D. Positioned in the left ventricular apex

E. Positioned on the wall of the right atrium near the entrance of the superior vena cava

29. Which of the following is *not* a constituent of the αβ T-cell receptor?

A. Constant region

B. Cytoplasmic tail

C. Disulphide bond
D. Kappa segment
E. Variable region

30. Which of the following statements regarding the spleen is *incorrect*?
    A. The spleen is a secondary lymphoid organ.
    B. The spleen is not a retroperitoneal organ.
    C. The spleen is supplied by afferent lymphatics.
    D. The spleen is supplied by the splenic artery.
    E. The spleen lies in the left upper quadrant of the abdomen.

31. Epithelium is defined by the expression of which adhesion molecule?
    A. E-cadherin
    B. E-selectin
    C. N-cadherin
    D. P-cadherin
    E. T-cadherin

32. What shape is the cartilage in the trachea?
    A. Continuous rings
    B. C-shaped
    C. Δ-(delta) shaped
    D. Ω-(omega) shaped
    E. None of the above

33. Sexual dysfunction is an adverse effect most associated with which of the following drugs?
    A. Lithium
    B. Monoamine oxidase inhibitors
    C. Noradrenaline and specific serotonergic antidepressants
    D. Serotonin–noradrenaline reuptake inhibitors
    E. Selective serotonin reuptake inhibitors

34. The axons of the ganglion cells enter the optic nerve via which of the following?
    A. Ciliary body
    B. Fovea centralis
    C. Macula lutea
    D. Optic bulb
    E. Optic papilla

35. How many types of cone are there with respect to spectral sensitivity?
    A. 2
    B. 3
    C. 4
    D. 5
    E. 6

36. Which of the following groups of muscles make up the rotator cuff?
    A. Latissimus dorsi, levator scapulae, teres minor, subscapularis
    B. Serratus anterior, teres minor, trapezius, subscapularis
    C. Supraspinatus, subclavius, subscapularis, teres minor
    D. Teres major, teres minor, deltoid, latissimus dorsi
    E. Teres minor, infraspinatus, supraspinatus, subscapularis

37. Which one of the following is *not* a function of antibodies?
    A. Activating complement
    B. Neutralizing toxins
    C. Presenting antigen to T-lymphocytes
    D. Preventing bacterial adhesion to tissue surfaces
    E. Promoting phagocytosis through opsonization

38. The region of an antigen to which an immunoglobulin molecule or cell surface receptor binds is known as the:
    A. Allotype
    B. Epitope
    C. Heavy chain
    D. Light chain
    E. Opsonin

39. In which part of the small intestine are Meckel diverticula usually found?
    A. Duodenum
    B. Ileum
    C. Jejunum
    D. All of the above
    E. None of the above

40. How many layers make up the retina?
    A. 4
    B. 5
    C. 6
    D. 7
    E. 8

41. Which of the following antianginal drugs is a potassium channel activator?
    A. Bisoprolol
    B. Diltiazem
    C. Glyceryl trinitrate
    D. Isosorbide mononitrate
    E. Nicorandil

42. Which one of the following cell types has no axonal process?
    A. Amacrine cells
    B. Cones

C. Ganglion cells
D. Horizontal cells
E. Rods

43. Which of the following forms an anastomosis between the superior and inferior mesenteric arteries?
    A. Ileocolic artery
    B. Left colic artery
    C. Marginal artery of Drummond
    D. Middle colic artery
    E. Right colic artery

44. Which one of the following is *not* part of a typical IgG antibody molecule?
    A. Disulphide bridges
    B. F_{ab}
    C. F_{bc}
    D. F_c
    E. Hypervariable regions

45. Which of the following best describes the location of the sinoatrial node?
    A. Has wide variability with regard to its position from person to person
    B. Positioned in the apical aspect of the right ventricle
    C. Positioned in the left atrial appendage
    D. Positioned in the right atrial septal wall
    E. Positioned on the wall of the right atrium near the entrance of the superior vena cava

46. Peptide YY is principally secreted by cells in which part of the small intestine?
    A. Duodenum
    B. Jejunum
    C. Proximal ileum
    D. Terminal ileum
    E. None of the above

47. The trachea is lined with which type of epithelium?
    A. Ciliated pseudostratified columnar
    B. Ciliated stratified columnar
    C. Simple columnar
    D. Simple squamous
    E. Stratified squamous

48. Which of the following nerve roots innervates the knee jerk (patellar tendon) reflex?
    A. L1, L2
    B. L2, L3
    C. L3, L4
    D. L4, L5
    E. L5, S1

49. Which type of muscle is trachealis?
   A. Cardiac
   B. Myotilin
   C. Skeletal
   D. Smooth
   E. None of the above

50. Which of the following drugs used in acute myocardial infarction should be adjusted for patients with renal impairment?
   A. Aspirin
   B. Clexane
   C. Clopidogrel
   D. Losartan
   E. Ramipril

Answers Paper 3

1. A – Abciximab
Abciximab is a chimeric monoclonal antibody which irreversibly binds GpIIb/IIIa receptors in platelets. This prevents the final common pathway of platelet aggregation. It is licensed for use in patients with unstable angina and non-ST elevation myocardial infarction who are undergoing primary coronary intervention. The term 'chimeric' refers to the fact that these antibodies are derived from DNA sources from more than one animal species (often mouse and human).

2. D – The posterior one-third of the tongue
The glossopharyngeal (IX) nerve originates from the medulla. It detects taste sensation from the posterior one-third of the tongue and also receives sensory information from the tonsils, pharynx and middle ear. Common pathologies include trauma, brainstem lesions and neck tumours. It is tested via the gag reflex.

3. E – Medial rotation of the shoulder
Teres major is a muscle of the posterior shoulder which is inserted on the anterior aspect of the humerus (medial side of the bicipital groove). It allows medial (or internal) rotation at the shoulder joint. It is also a shoulder adductor and is innervated by the lower subscapular nerve.

4. C – Femoral
The femoral artery is palpated at the groin by pressing the femoral artery against the inguinal ligament. The femoral artery travels through the groin in the femoral canal, accompanied by the femoral vein and femoral nerve.

5. D – Zonula occludens
Tight junctions (zonula occludens) are the areas in which cells are so closely joined together and they form virtually impermeable barriers. The major proteins which produce the tight junctions include claudins and occludins.

6. B – Type II collagen
Type II collagen is present in hyaline cartilage. It makes up to 50% of all proteins in cartilage. It forms a fibrillar network which supports the proteoglycan aggregate to provide tensile strength.

7. B – Fat transport
Lacteals are lymphatics within the small intestine that penetrate each villus to enable fat absorbed in the small intestine to be carried away into the lymphatic system.

8. D – Isosorbide mononitrate
Patients can rapidly develop tolerance to nitrates, such as isosorbide mononitrate. The probability of this happening can be reduced by ensuring that patients have an 8-hour period within 24 hours where they are free of nitrate treatment. Nitrates act by decreasing the preload by causing peripheral dilation. A decrease in the preload improves the cardiac output.

9. A – Hypercalcaemia
Digoxin is a cardiac glycoside extracted from the foxglove plant. It exerts its actions by inhibition of the Na^+/K^+ ATPase pump and decreases conduction through the atrioventricular node. Digoxin toxicity can be precipitated by hypokalaemia, hypomagnesemia and hypercalcaemia.

10. C – Squamous cell carcinoma
Squamous cell carcinoma is the most common type of laryngeal tumour, as the majority of the laryngeal epithelium is squamous. Verrucous carcinoma is a rare variant of squamous cell carcinoma which is linked to the use of snuff.

11. D – Hemidesmosome
Desmosomes promote cell-to-cell adhesion to help resist shearing forces. A costamere is a structural–functional component of striated muscle cells which join the force-generating sarcomeres to the sarcolemma. Hemidesmosomes are very small structures present on the inner basal surface of keratinocytes and act like desmosomes by forming spot junctions. The basal lamina is a layer of extracellular matrix upon which the epithelium sits.

12. E – Monocyte
A monocyte is an immigrant cell which will move to connective tissue when required to increase the macrophage population. A fibroblast synthesizes extracellular matrix and collagen. A macrophage (histiocyte) is fixed in connective tissue. A mast cell is also a resident cell.

13. A – C5
The trachea starts at the larynx which is level with the C5 vertebra. It continues until it bifurcates to become the primary bronchi at the T4/5 level.

14. A – Clozapine
Tardive dyskinesia manifests itself after long-term or high-dose antipsychotic use. While atypical antipsychotics are thought to be associated with a decreased risk of tardive dyskinesia, this association has only been demonstrated with clozapine.

15. C – Selective serotonin reuptake inhibitors
Selective serotonin reuptake inhibitors (SSRIs) are the safest antidepressant class when taken in overdose. This was reported in a study by

Isbister et al. who demonstrated that such agents are safer in an overdose despite serotonin syndrome being common. It was also concluded that citalopram was an exception to the rule, as it was associated with QTc prolongation.

16. D – Simvastatin

Statins can cause myositis and an elevated creatine kinase (CK) level. Patients initiated on treatment with statins should be warned of the side-effects and advised to discontinue use if they develop muscle pains or aching. It may be possible to try using a different statin; however, you may find that the patient is intolerant of all statins, and an alternative agent may need to be considered. Monitor the CK levels if they are elevated, along with the renal function.

17. A – Allopurinol

Enzyme inducers and inhibitors are common exam question topics. The liver enzyme inducers can decrease the effects of a number of drugs, including warfarin, and the enzyme inhibitors can increase the effects of drugs. Inhibition of the enzymes slows down the metabolism of drugs and therefore potentiates their effects. The enzyme inducers can be remembered by the mnemonic PC BRAS (Phenytoin, Carbamazepine, Barbiturates, Rifampicin, Alcohol [chronic excess], Sulphonylureas) and the inhibitors by AODEVICCES (Allopurinol, Omeprazole, Disulfiram, Erythromycin, Valproate, Isoniazid, Ciprofloxacin, Cimetidine, acute Ethanol intoxication, Sulphonamides).

18. E – Testicular artery

The testicular arteries are branches of the aorta. Embryologically, the testicles descend into the pelvis and retain their superior blood supply rather than gaining their supply from the internal iliac artery like the majority of the pelvic contents.

19. D – Paneth cells

Paneth cells are found throughout the intestinal tract, where they sit at the bottom of intestinal crypts. They contain zinc and lysozyme. They are thought to contribute to the host defence and regulation of intestinal flora. Enterocytes are the main cells of the intestine, goblet cells secrete mucous and stem cells are able to become any type of intestinal cell.

20. D – Zonula adherens

The zonula adherens (intermediate junctions) are the protein complexes which occur at cell-to-cell junctions. They appear as bands which encircle the cell. Cadherins are transmembrane proteins which bind cells together and are dependent upon calcium ions.

21. B – The aortic and pulmonary valves are tricuspid

The easiest way to remember this is that the mitral valve is the only one that is bicuspid. All of the other cardiac valves (aortic, pulmonary and tricuspid) have three valve leaflets. The tricuspid valve usually has three leaflets, although sometimes it may have two or four leaflets, and the number may change during its life. The most common form of congenital heart disease is a bicuspid aortic valve, and this occurs in approximately 1% of the population. Patients often present with aortic valve stenosis at the age of 40–60 years as a result of congenital bicuspid valves.

22. B – The adductor pollicis brevis
The muscles of the hand that are supplied by the median nerve can be remembered by the mnemonic 'LOAF':

- Lateral two lumbricals
- Opponens pollicis
- Abductor pollicis brevis
- Flexor pollicis brevis

The remainder are supplied by the ulnar nerve. Pronator teres is supplied by the median nerve and facilitates pronation of the forearm.

23. E – Ramipril
Patients with bilateral renal artery stenosis become dependent on the renin–angiotensin–aldosterone system in order to maintain renal perfusion. If either an angiotensin-converting enzyme (ACE) inhibitor or angiotensin-receptor blocker (ARB) is employed in the treatment of their hypertension, you will essentially complete a chemical nephrectomy. ACE inhibitors and ARBs can be used together, under strict guidance, for the treatment of heart failure and hypertension. Some large trials have shown particular benefit in combination treatment for patients with heart failure.

24. A – Fentanyl is a synthetic opioid commonly used in anaesthesia
Paracetamol is used to treat mild to moderate pain and is the first-line analgesic agent prescribed for simple tension headaches. Respiratory depression is an important side-effect of opioid use. Peptic ulceration is associated with non-steroidal anti-inflammatory drugs (NSAIDs), such as diclofenac and ibuprofen.

25. A – Pupillary constriction, drooping of eyelid and loss of sweating around the eye
Horner's syndrome describes a triad of signs which occur unilaterally: miosis (constricted pupil); partial ptosis (drooping of the eyelid); and loss of facial sweating (anhydrosis). Enophthalmos (posterior displacement of the eye) may also be present. Horner's syndrome is caused by an ipsilateral interruption of the sympathetic nerve supply to the eye.

26. A – The anterior two-thirds of the tongue
The facial nerve arises from the brainstem between the medulla and the pons. Its functions include the control of muscle of facial expression and taste sensation to the anterior two-thirds of the tongue. Pathology that affects the facial nerve include Bell's palsy, cerebello-pontine angle tumours, parotid tumours and herpes zoster infection.

27. B – The inferior gluteal nerve

The gluteus maximus is a muscle of the buttock region that acts to extend and rotate the thigh. It is supplied by the inferior gluteal nerve, derived from segments L5–S2. The obturator nerve supplies the adductors of the thigh, including the adductor longus, adductor magnus, adductor brevis and gracilis. The superior gluteal nerve innervates the abductors (gluteus medius, gluteus minimus and tensor fasciae latae). The sciatic nerve descends medial to psoas major and ultimately travels under gluteus maximus into the posterior compartment to supply the hamstrings. Finally, the femoral nerve supplies the quadriceps, as well as rectus femoris and pectineus.

28. A – Positioned between the atria and ventricles in the posteroinferior region of the interatrial septum, near the opening of the coronary sinus

The atrioventricular node (AVN) conducts electrical impulses received from the sinoatrial node. The AVN creates an important delay in conduction (usually 0.12 seconds), allowing atrial systole to occur prior to the ventricular systole. The AVN controls the rate at which ventricular contraction occurs and has an intrinsic firing rate of 40–60 beats per minute. The intrinsic rate becomes important in the context of deciphering heart blocks. The classic example is complete heart block, where there is complete atrioventricular dissociation. Here we see a ventricular rate (QRS complex) of between 40 and 60 beats per minute, and an atrial rate (P-waves) between 60 and 100 beats per minute. The P-waves are said to 'march through' the QRS complexes on the ECG.

29. D – Kappa segment

The most common form of T-cell receptor is the αβ T-cell receptor. It is a transmembrane receptor made up of two main subunits connected by disulphide bonds. Both subunits have cytoplasmic tails, a transmembranal region and extracellular hinge, constant and variable regions.

30. C – The spleen is supplied by afferent lymphatics

The spleen filters blood and traps blood-borne pathogens but has no role in filtering lymph. It therefore has no lymphatic supply or drainage. It is however a key secondary lymphoid organ. The spleen is suspended within its mesentery between the lienorenal ligament and gastrolienal ligament. The other statements in the question are true.

31. A – E-cadherin

Epithelial cadherin (E-cadherin) is a calcium-dependent cell-to-cell adhesion molecule. Loss of function is thought to contribute to the proliferation of cancer. E-cadherin downregulation decreases the strength of cellular adhesion within a tissue, allowing cells to cross the basement membrane and invade the surrounding tissue.

32. B – C-shaped

The trachea is comprised of 15–20 C-shaped cartilaginous rings which are able to reinforce the lateral and anterior sides of the airway. The posterior surface between the free ends of the cartilage is reinforced by the trachealis muscle.

33. E – Selective serotonin reuptake inhibitors

The effect of SSRIs on sexual function is still poorly understood. It has been hypothesized that the effects of serotonergic drugs on sexual function may relate to drug dose, serotonin receptor subtypes affected and the relative effect on serotonergic versus other receptors.

34. E – Optic papilla

The ganglion cells, which are found in the ganglion layer of the retina, enter the optic nerve via the optic papilla. This corresponds to a break in the visual field called the blind spot and is devoid of any light-sensitive rods or cones.

35. B – 3

Cones are specialized photosensitive receptors found in the retina and are capable of phototransduction. They function optimally in bright light and are mainly found in the central area of the retina. Cones allow colour perception and there are therefore three types: one sensitive to red, one sensitive to green and one sensitive to blue.

36. E – Teres minor, infraspinatus, supraspinatus, subscapularis

The rotator cuff protects the shallow glenohumeral joint, stabilizing the head of the humerus in the glenoid fossa. The supraspinatus abducts the humerus, while the other three muscles facilitate rotation. The infraspinatus and teres minor laterally rotate and adduct, while the subscapularis is responsible for medial rotation. The rotator cuff muscles can be remembered by the mnemonic 'SITS': Supraspinatus, Infraspinatus, Teres minor and Subscapularis.

37. C – Presenting antigen to T-lymphocytes

IgA in seromucous secretions has a particular role in preventing adhesion of bacteria to mucosal epithelia. Antibodies play a role in neutralizing bacterial toxins such as cholera and tetanus toxins. Complement binding to the F_c portion of the antibody activates complement through the classical pathway.

38. B – Epitope

The epitope is also known as antigenic determinant. The variable region of the F_{ab} (fragment antigen-binding) portion of an antibody is the region which has specificity to individual epitopes.

39. B – Ileum

In the fetus the ileum is connected to the umbilicus by the vitelline duct. If this duct fails to close, a Meckel diverticulum will persist. Meckel diverticula are present in approximately 2% of the population, located 2 feet from the ileocaecal valve, and are usually 2 inches in length. There are two types of ectopic tissue that may be found within these structures: gastric and pancreatic. Patients generally present at 2 years of age (e.g. with painless rectal bleeding or intussusception) and males are twice as likely to be affected.

40. E – 8
The retina is a light-sensitive tissue that lines the inner part of the eye. It is composed of eight layers: pigment; photoreceptor; outer nuclear; outer plexiform; inner nuclear; inner plexiform; ganglion cell; and nerve fibre. The retina also contains the optic disc where the ganglion cell axons leave the eye to form the optic nerve – this corresponds to the blind spot as it is devoid of photoreceptors.

41. E – Nicorandil
Nicorandil is a potassium channel activator and results in arterial vasodilation. It also has nitrate-like properties and promotes venous relaxation. Nicorandil can cause similar side-effects to nitrates, including headache, flushing, hypotension and dizziness. Patients should be started on small doses and titrated up to symptomatic relief.

42. A – Amacrine cells
Amacrine cells have no axons. They are octopus-like cells with dendrites emerging from one side. Amacrine cells are interneurons that regulate the bipolar cells and the ganglion cells in the retina. They are responsible for complex processing of the retinal image, specifically adjusting image brightness and, by integrating sequential activation of neurons, detecting motion.

43. C – Marginal artery of Drummond
The marginal artery of Drummond anastomoses the superior and inferior mesenteric arteries. It runs in the peritoneum and its absence should be considered an anatomic variant. The splenic flexure is approximately at the mid-point of the marginal artery and is the area most susceptible to watershed ischaemia.

44. C – F_{bc}
IgG antibodies are made up of two F_{ab} (fragment antigen-binding) regions and an F_c (fragment crystallizable) region connected by a hinge region. F_{ab} regions each have a hypervariable region at their distal end to which epitopes bind. Disulphide bridges are found in the hinge region and between the heavy and light chain components of the F_{ab} region.

45. E – Positioned on the wall of the right atrium near the entrance of the superior vena cava
The sinoatrial node (SAN) is a cluster of specialized cells often referred to as the primary pacemaker. These cells spontaneously generate electrical impulses and conduct an electrical charge resulting in atrial contraction.

There is subsequent electrical conduction to the atrioventricular node. The SAN has an intrinsic pacemaker rate of 60–100 beats per minute. Interruptions in the conduction of these electrical impulses can result in a variety of arrhythmias.

46. D – Terminal ileum
Peptide YY is secreted by the L-cells of the gastrointestinal mucosa. L-cells are principally found in the ileum and rectum, although they are present throughout the gastrointestinal tract. Peptide YY circulation increases postprandially and reduces intestinal motility, gallbladder contraction and pancreatic exocrine secretion. It also reduces appetite (i.e. is an ano-rectic) and is therefore thought to be a factor in energy homeostasis.

47. A – Ciliated pseudostratified columnar
The trachea is lined with ciliated pseudostratified columnar epithelium. The term 'pseudostratified' means that while there is only a single layer of cells, the nuclei of these cells are positioned similarly to stratified epithelia. The cilia act as one unit and beat rhythmically to remove mucous and irritants to prevent their descent further into the respiratory tract.

48. C – L3, L4
Striking the patella tendon with a tendon hammer causes passive stretching of the muscle which is detected by muscle spindles. Afferent signals from the muscle spindles travel via Ia nerve fibres. The α-motor neuron then carries efferent signals to facilitate contraction of rectus femoris, resulting in extension of the knee. Tendon reflexes form an integral part of the nervous system examination. Exaggerated reflexes occur in upper motor neuron lesions and in hyperthyroidism, while diminished reflexes occur in lower motor neuron lesions.

49. D – Smooth
Trachealis is a smooth muscle which attaches to the cartilaginous rings of the trachea. The function of this muscle is to allow constriction of the trachea. This constriction allows for a higher velocity of airflow in the trachea when coughing.

50. B – Clexane
Patients with ischaemic heart disease commonly have renovascular disease. Low molecular weight heparin (such as clexane [enoxaparin]), atenolol and digoxin may accumulate in severe renal failure due to poor excretion. Patients with a GFR <10 mL/min should have the dose of enoxaparin halved. Some even recommend that the dose be halved for those patients with a GFR <30 mL/min. Angiotensin-converting enzyme (ACE) inhibitors and angiotensin-receptor blockers should be used with extreme caution in patients with renal failure.

Questions Paper 4

1. The *RB1* tumour suppressor gene is located on which chromosome?
   A. 17p
   B. 5q
   C. 7q
   D. 13q
   E. 17q

2. At what vertebral level is the lower end of the conus medullaris found along the spinal cord?
   A. C1–C2
   B. L1–L2
   C. S1–S2
   D. T1–T2
   E. T11–T12

3. Which of the following is characteristic of a surgical third nerve (CN III) palsy in comparison to a medical cause?
   A. Disruption of the pupillary reflex
   B. Involvement of the facial nerve
   C. Spared pupillary involvement
   D. The eye facing down
   E. Unilateral ptosis

4. What is the correct order of a monosynaptic reflex arc?
   A. Afferent neuron, sensory receptor, integration centre, efferent neuron, muscle
   B. Muscle, efferent neuron, afferent neuron, integration centre, sensory receptor
   C. Muscle, sensory receptor, afferent neuron, integration centre, efferent neuron
   D. Sensory receptor, afferent neuron, integration centre, efferent neuron, muscle
   E. Sensory receptor, efferent neuron, integration centre, afferent neuron, muscle

5. Which of the following are polymers of tubulin?
   A. Actin filaments
   B. Intermediate filaments

C. Microtubules
D. All of the above
E. None of the above

6. Which one of the following is a non-organized type of gut-associated lymphoid tissue?
A. Cryptopatches
B. Intraepithelial lymphocytes
C. Isolated lymphoid follicles
D. Mesenteric lymph nodes
E. Peyer patches

7. To what is the filum terminale anchored?
A. The base of the skull
B. The clavicle
C. The coccyx
D. The L1 vertebrae
E. The ribs

8. Succinyl-CoA is formed by the action of which enzyme in the citric acid cycle?
A. Fumarate hydratase
B. Isocitrate dehydrogenase
C. Malate dehydrogenase
D. Oxoglutarate dehydrogenase
E. Succinate dehydrogenase

9. Where is the cauda equina found?
A. At the cervical section of the vertebral canal
B. At the L1–L2 section of the vertebral canal
C. At the T11–T12 level of the vertebral canal
D. In the cerebellum
E. In the cerebral cortex

10. The denticulate ligaments are:
A. Part of the arachnoid space
B. Part of the dura mater
C. Part of the dural space
D. Part of the pia mater
E. Part of the subarachnoid space

11. Which of the following is true of glycopeptide antibiotics?
A. They are active against Gram-negative organisms.
B. They are an example of a drug which has a low toxicity.
C. They are never nephrotoxic.
D. They inhibit peptidoglycan synthesis.
E. They penetrate into the cerebrospinal fluid.

12. Where is the fasciculus gracilis found?
    A. Lateral white columns
    B. Posterior grey columns
    C. Posterior lateral sulcus
    D. Posterior median sulcus
    E. Posterior white columns

13. Which layer of the gastrointestinal tract contains the Meissner's plexus?
    A. Mucosa
    B. Muscularis externa
    C. Muscularis mucosa
    D. Serosa
    E. Submucosa

14. In which layer of the gastrointestinal tract is the gut-associated lymphoid tissue primarily found?
    A. Mucosa
    B. Muscularis externa
    C. Muscularis mucosa
    D. Serosa
    E. Submucosa

15. Which type of tissue lines the oesophagus?
    A. Cuboidal epithelium
    B. Simple columnar epithelium
    C. Simple squamous epithelium
    D. Stratified squamous epithelium
    E. Transitional epithelium

16. The pylorus of the stomach is at which vertebral level?
    A. L1
    B. L2
    C. T10
    D. T11
    E. T12

17. During the conversion of isocitrate to oxoglutarate in the citric acid cycle, what is formed?
    A. NADH and CO_2
    B. NADH and H_2O
    C. NADPH and CO_2
    D. NADPH and CO_2 and H^+
    E. NADPH and H_2O

18. Which of the following is true of aminoglycoside antibiotics?
    A. They are always taken orally.
    B. They are ineffective against Gram-negative bacteria.

C. They are not ototoxic.

D. They inhibit the translocation of the peptidyl-tRNA.

E. They work by binding to the bacterial 60S ribosomal subunit.

19. Which four-carbon compound reacts with acetyl-CoA in the citric acid cycle?

A. Citrate

B. Oxaloacetate

C. Oxoglutarate

D. Pyruvate

E. Succinate

20. Which one of the following statements about the pulmonary pleura is *incorrect*?

A. Pleural reflections on each side meet at the angle of Louis.

B. The diaphragmatic pleura is innervated by the vagus nerve.

C. The parietal pleura is innervated by the intercostal nerves.

D. The pleural apex extends 2.5 cm above the clavicle.

E. Visceral pleura only has autonomic innervation.

21. Which is the outermost covering of the spinal cord?

A. Arachnoid mater

B. Dura mater

C. Pia mater

D. Subarachnoid space

E. Subdural space

22. Cardiac arrhythmias are *not* a common side-effect of which of the following electrolyte abnormalities?

A. Hyperkalaemia

B. Hypermagnesaemia

C. Hypokalaemia

D. Hypomagnesaemia

E. Hyponatraemia

23. Acetyl-CoA is formed by the conversion of what?

A. Acetylcholine

B. Acetyline-CoA

C. Glucose

D. Glycerol-3-phosphate

E. Pyruvate

24. A patient is found to be hypokalaemic postoperatively. Which of the following electrolytes, if also low, will need to be corrected within the plasma before the hypokalaemia will correctly resolve?

A. Bicarbonate

B. Calcium

C. Chloride

D. Magnesium
E. Sodium

25. Which one of the following can cause hypernatraemia?
    A. ACE inhibitor therapy in a patient with renal artery stenosis
    B. Excess use of 5% dextrose for IV fluid replacement
    C. High serum magnesium
    D. Multiple burns
    E. Syndrome of inappropriate ADH secretion

26. Following the transfusion of six units of blood, a patient's corrected calcium level was noted to be low. Why has this occurred?
    A. Citrate within blood products binds plasma calcium.
    B. Citrate within blood products results in increased calcium excretion.
    C. Excess potassium ions released from transfused cells are transported into cells along with calcium ions.
    D. Hypocalcaemia is likely to have resulted from deranged nutritional intake while critically ill in hospital.
    E. Transfused red blood cells contain albumin which binds plasma calcium.

27. A 53-year-old woman being treated for bipolar disorder develops hypothyroidism. What is the most likely offending drug?
    A. Amitriptyline
    B. Citalopram
    C. Fluoxetine
    D. Haloperidol
    E. Lithium

28. An elderly male patient presents to the emergency department in atrial fibrillation and is found to be hypokalaemic. If the patient was taking all of the below medications, which would you choose to discontinue first?
    A. Aspirin 75 mg od
    B. Bendroflumethiazide 2.5 mg od
    C. Cyclizine 50 mg tds
    D. Omeprazole 20 mg od
    E. Spironolactone 100 mg od

29. Which one of the following parts of the mitochondria contains adenosine triphosphate synthase?
    A. Crista
    B. Inner membrane
    C. Matrix
    D. Outer membrane
    E. Ribosome

30. Which of the following lesions causes internuclear ophthalmoplegia?
  A. A lateral longitudinal fasciculus lesion
  B. A medial longitudinal fasciculus lesion
  C. A trochlear nerve lesion
  D. An abducens nerve lesion
  E. An oculomotor nerve lesion

31. Which one of the following increases the surface area for chemical reactions within the mitochondria?
  A. Cristae
  B. Inner membrane
  C. Matrix
  D. Outer membrane
  E. Ribosome

32. Which one of the following is found in centrosomes?
  A. Alpha tubulin
  B. Beta tubulin
  C. Gamma tubulin
  D. All of the above
  E. None of the above

33. Which of the following medications is an absolute contraindication in pregnancy?
  A. Carbimazole
  B. Iodine
  C. Levothyroxine
  D. Propylthiouracil
  E. Radioiodine

34. Lid retraction is a clinical manifestation of hyperthyroidism. What causes this and which drug may be used to treat it?
  A. Parasympathetic overactivity of smooth muscle; carbimazole
  B. Parasympathetic overactivity of smooth muscle; levothyroxine
  C. Parasympathetic over-innervation of skeletal muscle; levothyroxine
  D. Sympathetic overactivity of smooth muscle; carbimazole
  E. Sympathetic over-innervation of skeletal muscle; carbimazole

35. Patients should be advised to seek immediate medical advice if they experience symptoms such as sore throat, fever, mouth ulcers and bleeding when taking which drug?
  A. Carbimazole
  B. Iodine
  C. Levothyroxine
  D. Liothyronine
  E. Propranolol

36. Which of the following classes of antibiotic is most effective against Gram-negative sepsis?
    A. Aminoglycosides
    B. Macrolides
    C. Oxazolidinones
    D. Penicillins
    E. Tetracyclines

37. Combination drug co-trimoxazole is:
    A. Effective at 1/10 of the dose of what would be needed if given separately
    B. Effective at 1/1000 of the dose of what would be needed if given separately
    C. Known to have no effect on folate synthesis
    D. Known to potentiate the action of tinzaparin
    E. Less effective than when given separately

38. Clindamycin is a type of which antibiotic group?
    A. Fluoroquinolones
    B. Lincosamides
    C. Macrolides
    D. Penicillins
    E. Tetracyclines

39. Which of the following is the most common cause of an acute upper respiratory infection?
    A. Bacteria
    B. Fungi
    C. Parasite
    D. Virus
    E. None of the above

40. Which of the following is the most common cause of an upper respiratory tract infection?
    A. Adenovirus
    B. Influenza virus
    C. Parainfluenza virus
    D. Respiratory syncytial virus
    E. Rhinovirus

41. Which of the following is *not* a cause of peripheral cyanosis?
    A. Deep vein thrombosis
    B. Hypothermia
    C. Hypovolaemia
    D. Polycythaemia rubra vera
    E. Raynaud phenomenon

42. What kind of hearing deficit is most frequently produced by an acoustic neuroma?
    A. Asymmetrical hearing loss
    B. Balance problems
    C. Complete hearing loss
    D. Progressive tinnitus
    E. Vertigo

43. Which of the following is characteristic of a paralytic squint but is *not* a feature of a non-paralytic squint?
    A. It is always convergent
    B. It is always divergent
    C. It is an acquired condition
    D. It is associated with diplopia
    E. It is present from birth

44. The Ras proto-oncogene is mutated in what percentage of human cancers?
    A. 10%
    B. 25%
    C. 40%
    D. 50%
    E. 75%

45. Which one of the following is *not* a cause of hyperkalaemia?
    A. Addison disease
    B. Conn syndrome
    C. Massive blood transfusion
    D. Metabolic acidosis
    E. Rhabdomyolysis

46. The *Ras* gene codes for which protein?
    A. ATPase proteins
    B. Epidermal growth factor receptor
    C. GTPase proteins
    D. Platelet-derived growth factor
    E. Vascular endothelial growth factor

47. Which of the following conditions causes a degeneration of retinal ganglion cells?
    A. Glaucoma
    B. Leber hereditary optic neuropathy
    C. Meningioma
    D. Parkinson's disease
    E. Retinitis

48. Which of the following causes a sensorineural hearing impairment as opposed to conductive deficit?
   A. Foreign body
   B. Long QT syndrome
   C. Ménière disease
   D. Pendred syndrome
   E. Wax

49. Mutation in the *Ras* gene produces a protein that:
   A. Codes for the epidermal growth factor receptor
   B. Codes for the platelet-derived growth factor
   C. Codes for the vascular endothelial growth factor
   D. Is always active
   E. Is not active

50. What molecule is fumarate converted to in the citric acid cycle?
   A. Malate
   B. Oxaloacetate
   C. Oxoglutarate
   D. Pyruvate
   E. Succinate

Answers Paper 4

1. D – 13q
The *RB1* (retinoblastoma) gene is implicated in causing the rare eye cancer retinoblastoma. The *RB1* gene can be found on chromosome 13q. In hereditary retinoblastoma, sufferers are born with one defective RB1 allele. A mutation then occurs on the remaining good allele, resulting in two defective copies of the gene. This results in the formation of retinoblastoma. These are rare eye tumours usually affecting children under 5 years of age.

2. B – L1–L2
The conus medullaris is at the terminal end of the spinal cord, at the vertebral level L1/2. The upper end of the conus medullaris is not usually well defined.

3. A – Disruption of the pupillary reflex
Third nerve palsies without pupil dilation are characteristic of a medical cause, such as diabetes or giant cell arthritis. On the other hand, early dilation of the pupil associated with the palsy is suggestive of a compressive or 'surgical' cause as the parasympathetic fibres, which are involved in the papillary reflex, run on the outer aspect of the nerve.

4. D – Sensory receptor, afferent neuron, integration centre, efferent neuron, muscle
The receptor at the end of a sensory neuron reacts to a stimulus. The afferent neuron conducts nerve impulses along an afferent pathway towards the central nervous system. The integration centre consists of one or more synapses in the central nervous system. The efferent neuron conducts a nerve impulse along an efferent pathway from the integration centre to an effector. Where the effector is a skeletal muscle, it responds to the efferent impulses by contracting.

5. C – Microtubules
Microtubules are polymers of tubulin and are usually made from 13 tubulin monomers. Elongation occurs at the positive end of the polymer. Actin is the monomer subunit of microfilaments and thin filaments, and intermediate filaments produce a dimer which is formed through the coiling of two monomers.

6. B – Intraepithelial lymphocytes

Non-organized gut-associated lymphoid tissue (GALT) includes intraepithelial lymphocytes and lamina propria lymphocytes. Organized GALTs are cryptopatches, Peyer patches, isolated lymphoid follicles and mesenteric lymph nodes. GALT generates lymphoid cells and antibodies. It is a type of mucosa-associated lymphoid tissue (MALT).

7. C – The coccyx

The filum terminale (terminal thread) is the fibrous extension of the pia mater from the apex of the conus medullaris. It consists of two parts. The upper part reaches the lower border of the second sacral vertebrae. It is surrounded by the nerves which form the cauda equina. The lower part is closely adherent to the dura mater and is attached to the posterior aspect of the first segment of the coccyx. It is also known as the coccygeal ligament.

8. D – Oxoglutarate dehydrogenase

Oxoglutarate is a five-carbon compound. It is metabolized by the enzyme oxoglutarate dehydrogenase to form succinyl-CoA. During the conversion of oxoglutarate to succinyl-CoA, one molecule of NADH and one molecule of CO_2 are formed. Succinyl-CoA is acted on by the enzyme succinyl-CoA synthetase to form succinate. During the conversion of succinyl-CoA to succinate, a molecule of guanosine triphosphate (GTP) is formed as well as a molecule of coenzyme A (CoA). These are also removed from the cycle. The four-carbon molecule succinate is further metabolized by the enzyme succinate dehydrogenase to form another four-carbon compound, fumarate. During the conversion of succinate to fumarate, two hydrogen ions and two electrons are formed; these two electrons enter the electron transport chain.

9. B – At the L1–L2 section of the vertebral canal

The cauda equina is a collection of nerve roots at the inferior end of the vertebral canal at approximately L1–L2. It comes to an end at this level as while the spinal cord halts growth in infancy, the bones of the spine continue to grow. There is some positional variation in adults. Lumbar punctures are therefore performed at the L3/4 vertebral level to prevent complications secondary to spinal cord trauma.

10. D – Part of the pia mater

The paired denticulate ligaments of the pia mater attach the spinal cord to the arachnoid and dura mater at 21 positions on each side. They are important in providing stability to the spinal cord by preventing motion within the vertebral column.

11. D – They inhibit peptidoglycan synthesis

Vancomycin is an example of a glycopeptide antibiotic that inhibits peptidoglycan synthesis. Glycopeptide antibiotics are toxic (particularly nephrotoxic), are ineffective against Gram-negative organisms and, while they are bacteriostatic against most species, they are only bacteri-cidal against enterococci. They will not penetrate into the cerebrospinal fluid.

12. E – Posterior white columns
The fasciculus gracilis (or tract of Goll) is the bundle of axonal fibres which carries information about fine touch, vibration and conscious pro-prioception from the lower part of the body to the brain stem. It is found in the posterior white columns (or the dorsal column–medial lemniscus pathway). More specifically, the fasciculus gracilis is found medially and the fasciculus cuneatus is found laterally. It increases in size as the col-umn moves upwards, as it collects and carries more fibres.

13. E – Submucosa
Meissner's plexus (submucosal plexus) is found within the submucosa and is formed by the branches which come from the myenteric plexus and have perforated the circular muscle fibres. They innervate cells within the epithelium and the smooth muscle layer. It only contains parasympathetic fibres, in contrast to Auerbach's plexus which carries both sympathetic and parasympathetic innervation.

14. A – Mucosa
The mucosa is the innermost layer of the gastrointestinal tract. Gut-associated lymphoid tissue (GALT) is the digestive tract's immune sys-tem and is primarily found in the mucosa, although it sometimes extends into the submucosa. The submucosa comprise dense irregular connec-tive tissue. Within the submucosa are the lymphatic vessels and nerve plexuses. Meissner's plexus is located in the submucosa. The muscularis externa consists of thick layers of smooth muscle. The myenteric plexus of Auerbach is located in the muscularis externa.

15. D – Stratified squamous epithelium
The oesophagus is lined with non-keratinizing stratified squamous epi-thelium. These are flat (squamous) scale-like cells which are layered (stratified) but not keratinized. It allows some resistance to extremes of temperature and texture. Simple epithelia have only one layer.

16. A – L1
The pylorus of the stomach (a strong ring of smooth muscle) is at the level of L1 in the transpyloric plane (of Addison) and is generally on the right side. It is the connection between the distal stomach and the duodenum.

17. A – NADH and CO_2
The six-carbon molecule of isocitrate is acted on by the enzyme isocitrate dehydrogenase to form the five-carbon compound oxoglutarate. During the conversion of isocitrate to oxoglutarate, one molecule of NADH and one molecule of CO_2 are formed.

18. D – They inhibit the translocation of the peptidyl-tRNA
Aminoglycoside antibiotics work by binding to the bacterial 30S ribosomal subunit which inhibits the translocation of the peptidyl-tRNA from the A-site to the P-site. This means the bacterium is unable to synthesize proteins vital to its growth. They are ototoxic and nephrotoxic. They are effective against Gram-positive and Gram-negative bacteria. They are never administered orally but through intramuscular or intravenous injection.

19. B – Oxaloacetate
Oxaloacetate is a four-carbon molecule. It reacts with a two-carbon molecule of acetyl-CoA to form the six-carbon compound citrate. At this point in the citric acid cycle, one molecule of carbon dioxide is removed to form the five-carbon compound oxoglutarate. Another carbon dioxide molecule is removed at this point to form the four-carbon compound succinate, which is converted via oxidation back into oxaloacetate so that it can be reused in another iteration of the citric acid cycle.

20. B – The diaphragmatic pleura is innervated by the vagus nerve
The diaphragmatic pleura is innervated by the phrenic nerve. The visceral pleura only has the autonomic innervations of the vagus nerve and perceives stretch but not pain. Both visceral and diaphragmatic pleurae are receptive to pain.

21. B – Dura mater
There are three layers covering the spinal cord. From outermost to innermost, they are the dura mater, arachnoid mater and pia mater.

22. E – Hyponatraemia
Potassium and magnesium are both intracellular ions required for adequate cardiac cell functioning and stabilization of the cardiac cell membrane. Increases or decreases in these ions make cardiac cells more vulnerable to abnormal function, and therefore electrical disturbance, resulting in life-threatening arrhythmias.

23. E – Pyruvate
Pyruvate is metabolized by pyruvate dehydrogenase to form acetyl-CoA. Pyruvate can also be acted on by another enzyme, pyruvate carboxylase, to form oxaloacetate, which is an important intermediary in the tricyclic acid (TCA) cycle. Acetyl-CoA is a two-carbon compound that binds with the four-carbon compound oxaloacetate, via citrate synthase, to form citrate. Citrate is then metabolized by the enzyme aconitase to an intermediate compound called *cis*-aconitate by removing a water molecule. *cis*-Aconitate is further metabolized by the enzyme aconitase and is converted to isocitrate by adding a water molecule. Isocitrate is still a six-carbon compound but it has been structurally altered by the removal and addition of a water molecule. Isocitrate is converted into the five-carbon compound oxoglutarate by the enzyme isocitrate dehydrogenase.

During the conversion of isocitrate to oxoglutarate, one molecule of NADH and one molecule of CO_2 are formed.

24. D – Magnesium
Potassium channels are inhibited by magnesium. When plasma levels of magnesium are low, a higher concentration of potassium moves into the extracellular spaces and is subsequently excreted by the kidneys.

25. D – Multiple burns
Any condition causing the excess loss of water in comparison to sodium (e.g. burns, diarrhoea) will result in hypernatraemia, as will excessive use of NaCl for IV fluid replacement. Overuse of IV dextrose fluid use and SIADH will decrease plasma levels of sodium. ACE inhibitor medication in patients with renal artery stenosis can result in acute renal failure, producing hyperkalaemia but not hypernatraemia.

26. A – Citrate within blood products binds plasma calcium
Citrate is contained within blood products in order to prevent coagulation. This binds to calcium, resulting in hypocalcaemia. Transfused red blood cells do not contain albumin. If a patient was hypocalcaemic from low dietary intake, assuming adequate parathyroid function, increases in parathyroid hormone levels would stimulate calcium resorption from bone to correct this.

27. E – Lithium
Lithium is used in the treatment of bipolar disorder and depression. One must be aware of its numerous side-effects including toxicity to the thyroid gland, which may result in the development of hypothyroidism. It is therefore recommended that patients taking lithium have regular check-ups to monitor for symptoms of hypothyroidism as well as blood tests for thyroid status monitoring.

28. B – Bendroflumethiazide 2.5 mg od
Thiazide diuretics (and other non–potassium-sparing diuretics) are a common cause of hypokalaemia within the elderly population being treated for hypertension and cardiac failure. Stopping omeprazole and aspirin would have no effect on plasma potassium. The patient may be taking cyclizine to prevent persistent vomiting, which could be the cause of his hyponatraemia. Spironolactone is an aldosterone antagonist and therefore is potassium-sparing.

29. B – Inner membrane
ATP synthase is found in the inner membrane of mitochondria to allow for the generation of ATP in the matrix.

30. B – A medial longitudinal fasciculus lesion
Damage to the medial longitudinal fasciculus causes internuclear ophthalmoplegia. This is characterized by weakness in adduction of the

ipsilateral eye with nystagmus on abducting the contralateral eye. It is classically seen in multiple sclerosis.

31. A – Cristae
Cristae are the internal folds formed by the inner membrane of mitochondria. They allow an increased surface area for aerobic respiration to take place. For example, the inner membranes of hepatic mitochondria have five times the active area when compared to the outer membranes.

32. C – Gamma tubulin
Gamma tubulin is found in centrosomes and acts as a nucleating site for microtubule assembly. α- and β-tubulin become dimers and are assembled to form microtubules.

33. E – Radioiodine
Radioiodine is an absolute contraindication in pregnancy. The other drugs listed are all safe but must be used with caution in pregnancy. Carbimazole and propylthiouracil should be used with the lowest dose possible to control symptoms, as they both may cross the placenta and therefore high levels may cause fetal hypothyroidism.

34. D – Sympathetic overactivity of smooth muscle; carbimazole
Sympathetic overactivity of smooth muscle causes lid retraction and proptosis (anterior bulging of the eye) in hyperthyroidism. Proptosis may prevent the eyes from closing properly, which can cause corneal scarring and oedematous conjunctiva. Carbimazole should be used first as this treats the underlying cause of hyperthyroidism. Topical treatments for immediate symptomatic relief may also be administered, e.g. lubricating eye drops or steroids to help reduce inflammation.

35. A – Carbimazole
Agranulocytosis is a rare toxic side-effect of carbimazole therapy. Before therapy is commenced, patients should be advised to stop the drug and seek medical advice if any symptoms such as fever, sore throat or mouth ulceration occur. Eventually, serious systemic infections can arise due to lack of neutrophils, causing a compromise in immunological defence. Propylthiouracil can be initiated instead, although symptoms may still arise with this medication and therefore similar advice should be given when starting this drug.

36. A – Aminoglycosides
Aminoglycosides, such as gentamicin, are useful in treating Gram-negative sepsis. Tetracyclines and macrolides are effective against Gram-negative bacteria but not as effective as an aminoglycoside during sepsis. Oxazolidinones and penicillins are not effective against Gram-negative bacteria.

37. A – Effective at 1/10 of the dose of what would be needed if given separately

Sulphamethoxazole and trimethoprim combine to form co-trimoxazole. The sulphonamide part of the drug acts against folate synthesis at an earlier stage than most other antibiotics. Therefore, when in combination, the drugs are effective at 1/10 of what would be needed if each drug was given on its own.

38. B – Lincosamides

Lincosamides, such as clindamycin, are active against Gram-positive cocci. They inhibit protein synthesis in bacterial cells only by disrupting ribosomal activity. Use clindamycin with care, as its most severe common side-effect is *Clostridium difficile*-associated diarrhoea.

39. D – Virus

Viral upper respiratory tract infections (URTIs) are the most common. Species such as rhinovirus, parainfluenza virus, coronavirus, adenovirus, respiratory syncytial virus and the influenza virus account for most causes. Hence for most causes of true URTIs, antibiotics will be contraindicated.

40. E – Rhinovirus

Rhinovirus is the most common causative viral infective agent of an URTI. It is a single-stranded RNA virus and is implicated in up to 50% of URTIs.

41. D – Polycythaemia rubra vera

Polycythaemia rubra vera is a myeloproliferative disorder, commonly associated with erythroid hyperplasia, thrombocytosis and splenomegaly. Patients initially present with plethora but can present uncommonly with erythematous, warm or painful burning distal extremities.

42. A – Asymmetrical hearing loss

An acoustic neuroma is a benign schwannoma of the vestibular nerve that presents with an asymmetrical loss of hearing and vertigo presenting later in the course of disease. With progression, ipsilateral cranial nerves V, VI, IX, and X may become involved. They present bilaterally in type II neurofibromatosis and account for 80% of cerebello-pontine angle tumours.

43. C – It is an acquired condition

A paralytic squint (or incomitant strabismus) is an acquired defect that is said to exist when the angle of the deviation varies with the direction of gaze. When the normal eye is fixing on an object, the degree of strabismus shown by the other eye is termed 'primary' deviation. When the abnormal eye is fixing, the angle of squint is greater and is referred to as 'secondary' deviation.

44. D – 50%

The Ras proto-oncogene is mutated in approximately one out of four human cancers (25%). The *Ras* gene is a family of genes which encode small GTPases that are involved in cellular signal transduction. Activation of Ras signalling promotes cell growth, differentiation and cell survival. Ras communicates signals from outside the cell to the nucleus, and mutations in *Ras* genes can result in permanent activation. This results in inappropriate transmission inside the cell. Because these signals lead to cell growth and division, dysregulated Ras signalling can lead to oncogenesis and tumour formation.

45. B – Conn syndrome
Conn syndrome is primary hyperaldosteronism (i.e. occurs independent of the renin–angiotensin system). Aldosterone acts within the kidney to retain sodium at the expense of potassium, therefore hyperaldosteronism causes hypokalaemia. Addison disease is caused by destruction or dysfunction of the adrenal cortex. This reduces the amount of aldosterone produced and secreted, resulting in hyperkalaemia. Because potassium is an intracellular cation, any process causing cell destruction (e.g. rhabdomyolysis, lysis of stored red blood cells for transfusion) will release excess potassium into the plasma. In acidosis, excess H^+ ions are transported into the cells in exchange for K^+ ions, which therefore increase K^+ ion concentration within the plasma.

46. C – GTPase proteins
The *Ras* gene codes for GTPase proteins. GTPase proteins transmit signals from the cell surface growth factor receptors. Activation of Ras signalling causes cell growth, differentiation and survival. Mutation in *Ras* genes can cause permanent activation resulting in uncontrolled cell growth and differentiation, and as such can lead to tumour formation.

47. B – Leber hereditary optic neuropathy
Leber hereditary optic neuropathy (LHON) is a mitochondrial inherited disorder that leads to the degeneration of retinal ganglion cells. It mainly affects young men and presents with acute-onset visual loss in first one eye, and then the other.

48. C – Ménière disease
Ménière disease causes a sensorineural hearing impairment. It presents with recurrent attacks of vertigo, fluctuating sensorineural hearing impairment and tinnitus, and is caused by endolymphatic hydrops. It is treated with rest, reassurance and antihistamines. In severe cases, endolymphatic sac surgery or ablation of the vestibular organ may be considered.

49. D – Is always active
Mutations in the *Ras* gene produce a protein that is always active, even when there is no stimulating signal from growth factor receptors. This results in cell proliferation that is uncontrolled.

50. A – Malate

Fumarate is a four-carbon compound and is an intermediary molecule in the citric acid cycle. Fumarate is acted on by fumarate hydratase to form a four-carbon compound malate. During this reaction, a water molecule is added. Malate is metabolized by the enzyme malate dehydrogenase into oxaloacetate. During the conversion of malate to oxaloacetate, a molecule of NADH is formed. Oxaloacetate is a four-carbon compound and is combined with acetyl-CoA via the enzyme citrate synthase to form the six-carbon compound citrate.

Questions Paper 5

1. Which part of a blood vessel plays a key role in mediating chemical signals which control vascular tone?
   A. Adventitia
   B. Elastica interna
   C. Endothelium
   D. Intima
   E. Media

2. Which one of the following statements regarding lymphocytes is true?
   A. B-lymphocytes function by acting directly against virus-infected cells and tumour cells
   B. B-lymphocytes give rise to plasma cells
   C. B-lymphocytes produce plasma cells, which produce antigens
   D. Lymphocytes are found mainly in the plasma
   E. T-lymphocytes give rise to plasma cells

3. The activation of C3 by C3 convertase can occur via three pathways. Which of the following pathways below describes activation via antibody binding to bacteria?
   A. Alternative pathway
   B. Apoptosis
   C. Classical pathway
   D. Lectin pathway
   E. Tyrosine kinase pathway

4. Which one of the following is responsible for knee flexion and ankle plantar flexion?
   A. Biceps femoris
   B. Gastrocnemius
   C. Popliteus
   D. Rectus femoris
   E. Tibialis anterior

5. How many pairs of cervical nerves are there in the human spinal cord?
   A. 7
   B. 8
   C. 9
   D. 10
   E. 11

6. Which of the following initiates the process of platelet aggregation?
   A. Activation of platelets and subsequent generation of arachidonic acid and synthesis of thromboxane A2
   B. Adhesion of platelets to thrombogenic surfaces
   C. Exposure of vessel wall collagen
   D. Expression of glycoprotein IIb/IIIa receptors
   E. Platelet aggregation with fibrinogen binding to glycoprotein IIb/IIIa

7. Penicillins belong to which group of antibiotics?
   A. Aminoglycosides
   B. β-Lactams
   C. Carbapenems
   D. Lincosamides
   E. Tetracyclines

8. Which one of the following statements is true regarding vitamin B_{12} therapy?
   A. Vitamin B_{12} can only be administered orally.
   B. Vitamin B_{12} is indicated for the treatment of anaemia of chronic renal failure.
   C. Vitamin B_{12} is indicated for the treatment of pernicious anaemia.
   D. Vitamin B_{12} is not required for DNA synthesis.
   E. Vitamin B_{12} treatment requires regular weekly injections for life.

9. Which one of the following blocks calcium channels directly, inhibiting the influx of Ca^{2+} into smooth muscle cells?
   A. Amlodipine
   B. Diazoxide
   C. Doxazosin
   D. Glyceryl trinitrate
   E. Ramipril

10. Which one of the following major vessels consistently carries deoxygenated blood?
    A. Ascending aorta
    B. Brachiocephalic trunk
    C. Pulmonary artery
    D. Pulmonary vein
    E. Thoracic aorta

11. Which one of the following statements is true regarding the drug aspirin?
    A. Aspirin activates antithrombin III, which limits blood clotting by inactivating thrombin and factor X.
    B. Aspirin inhibits platelet aggregation.
    C. Aspirin is an antifibrinolytic agent.

D. Aspirin is originally derived from the rubber plant.
E. Aspirin is recommended as an analgesic in children less than 12 years of age.

12. Which of the following vein anastomoses with the azygous system of veins?
    A. Hepatic vein
    B. Left gastric vein
    C. Portal vein
    D. Splenic vein
    E. Superior mesenteric

13. Phagocytosis requires the attachment of a phagocyte to an offending organism. One way this is done is via opsonization. Which one of the following does *not* act as an opsonin?
    A. Collectin
    B. Complement
    C. E-selectin
    D. IgA
    E. IgG

14. Which of the following vessels carries blood from the liver into the inferior vena cava?
    A. Hepatic vein
    B. Left gastric vein
    C. Portal vein
    D. Splenic vein
    E. Superior mesenteric

15. Which of the following vessels' tone is the principal determinant of systemic vascular resistance?
    A. Arteriole
    B. Artery
    C. Capillary
    D. Vein
    E. Venule

16. Which one of the following statements is most accurate regarding folic acid?
    A. Folate deficiency results in microcytic anaemia.
    B. Folate is not required for DNA synthesis.
    C. Folic acid is administered by intramuscular injections.
    D. Folic acid supplements are associated with many unpleasant side-effects.
    E. Since the introduction of folic acid supplements for pregnant women, the rate of neural tube defects in newborn babies has fallen markedly.

17. Tetracyclines affect which part of a bacterium?
    A. They cause anticodon recognition which leads to the misreading of DNA.
    B. They cause premature termination of the peptide chain.
    C. They compete with tRNA for the A-site.
    D. They inhibit translocation.
    E. They inhibit transpeptidation.

18. Which one of the following classes of antimicrobial inhibits DNA topoisomerase II?
    A. Aminoglycosides
    B. Fluoroquinolones
    C. Lincosamides
    D. Macrolides
    E. Penicillins

19. Which one of the following statements regarding iron is true?
    A. Approximately 25% of the body's iron supply is in haemoglobin.
    B. In the blood, iron is transported loosely bound to a transport protein called ferritin.
    C. Iron is stored inside cells as protein–iron complexes such as transferrin and haemosiderin.
    D. Small amounts of iron are lost each day in urine and perspiration.
    E. The average daily loss of iron is 1 mg in women and men.

20. Ethambutol is effective against which of the following organisms?
    A. *Haemophilus*
    B. *Mycobacterium*
    C. *Neisseria*
    D. *Staphylococcus*
    E. *Streptococcus*

21. Which of the following classes of biochemical reactions is the best target for chemotherapy?
    A. Class I
    B. Class II
    C. Class III
    D. Class IV
    E. Class V

22. Which one of the following antibiotics inhibits folate synthesis?
    A. Aminoglycosides
    B. Lincosamides
    C. Penicillins
    D. Sulphonamides
    E. Tetracyclines

23. Which of the following statements regarding thalassaemias is true?
    A. It is associated with a reduced risk of infection.
    B. It is caused by absent or faulty alpha and beta globin chains.
    C. It is caused by absent or faulty alpha or beta globin chains.
    D. It is typically seen in people of North European ancestry.
    E. Sickle cell anaemia is one of the many variants of thalassaemia.

24. Which one of the following is a β-lactamase inhibitor?
    A. Benzylpenicillin
    B. Ciprofloxacin
    C. Clavulanic acid
    D. Clindamycin
    E. Piperacillin

25. Opsonization is mediated by which of the following components of the complement cascade?
    A. C3a
    B. C3b
    C. C5a
    D. C6
    E. C7

26. Which one of the following statements regarding the vasculature of the kidney is correct?
    A. The arterial supply of the kidneys arises via one common renal artery which branches from the abdominal aorta.
    B. The kidneys are supplied by branches of the coeliac artery.
    C. The paired renal arteries arise from the abdominal aorta beneath the inferior mesenteric artery.
    D. The renal arteries subdivide to form interlobar, arcuate and interlobular arteries.
    E. The right renal vein receives the right gonadal vein before draining to the inferior vena cava.

27. In order to induce osmotic cell lysis, the terminal components of the complement cascade produce:
    A. A membrane attack complex
    B. Elastase enzyme
    C. Hydrogen peroxide
    D. Lipopolysaccharide
    E. Reactive oxygen species

28. Which of the following classes of drug prevents the negative supercoiling of DNA?
    A. Aminoglycosides
    B. Fluoroquinolones
    C. Lincosamides

D. Macrolides

E. Penicillins

29. Which components of the complement cascade are known as anaphyla-toxins due to their ability to induce histamine release by mast cells, and thereby vasodilation?

A. C3a and C5a

B. C3b and C5b

C. C6 and C7

D. C6 and C9

E. C7 and C9

30. Which of the following statements is *not* true regarding folic acid deficiency anaemia?

A. In the bone marrow it causes a form of megaloblastic anaemia.

B. It is associated with neurological damage.

C. It commonly occurs in dietary deficiency.

D. It may be due to alcoholism.

E. It may be due to coeliac disease.

31. Complications of vitamin B_{12} deficiency include all of the following *except*:

A. Breathlessness

B. Glossitis

C. Pernicious anaemia

D. Reduced myelin production in the spinal cord

E. Reversible neurological damage

32. Avascular necrosis most commonly occurs at which anatomical location?

A. Anterior superior iliac spine

B. Femoral head

C. Head of the fifth metatarsal

D. Maxillary process

E. Mid-shaft of the humerus

33. Which one of the following statements about human haemoglobin is *not* true?

A. Carbon dioxide complexes with haemoglobin to form carboxyhaemoglobin

B. Each haem group bears an atom of iron.

C. Haemoglobin does not exist freely in the plasma.

D. Normal values for haemoglobin are 13–18 g/100 mL in an adult male.

E. The globin part of the haemoglobin molecule consists of four poly-peptide chains.

34. Regarding the composition of plasma, which one of the following is correct?

A. Albumin accounts for 36% of plasma proteins.

B. Fibrinogen accounts for 14% of plasma proteins.

C. Globulins contribute to 60% of the plasma proteins.

D. Plasma proteins carry thyroid hormones.

E. Water contributes to 10% of the total plasma volume.

35. Which one of the following electrolytes is found at higher concentrations within the extracellular fluid compared to the intracellular fluid?

A. Ca^{2+}

B. K^+

C. Mg^{2+}

D. Na^+

E. PC_4^{2-}

36. Which one of the following statements with regard to basophils is true?

A. Basophils are the most common white blood cell.

B. Basophils bind specifically to immunoglobulin A.

C. The most important role of basophils is to lead the counterattack against parasitic worms.

D. Their nucleus contains histamine granules.

E. Stained basophils have U-shaped nuclei.

37. Which one of the following is the narrowest part of the male urethra?

A. Membranous urethra

B. Preprostatic (intramural) urethra

C. Prostatic urethra

D. Proximal urethra

E. Spongy urethra

38. Which of the following statements about the secretion of vasopressin is correct?

A. A decrease in plasma volume will cause an indirect inhibition of vasopressin release.

B. Osmoreceptors within the brainstem detect changes in plasma osmo-lality and cause release of vasopressin.

C. Oxytocin and vasopressin are synthesized within the cell body of the same neurons.

D. Vasopressin is secreted from the anterior pituitary gland.

E. Vasopressin release is stimulated by an increase in plasma osmolality.

39. Which one of the following statements describing erythropoietin is *incorrect*?

A. Blood-borne erythropoietin stimulates the spleen to produce more erythrocytes.

B. Erythropoietin is a glycoprotein hormone.

C. Erythropoietin is produced by the liver and kidneys.

D. Hypoxia stimulates the production of erythropoietin.

E. People living at higher altitudes have increased rates of erythropoietin production.

40. Regarding body water and its distribution, which of the following statements is correct?
    A. Approximately two-thirds of total body water is intracellular.
    B. At least 90% of an infant's body mass is composed of water.
    C. Extracellular fluid is located primarily within the intravascular and interstitial spaces, the majority of which is contained within the intravascular plasma.
    D. Females have a higher percentage of body water in comparison to males.
    E. The average person's plasma volume is 6 L.

41. A cross section through a particular point of the spinal cord shows a larger grey matter (butterfly) area compared with the white mater. At which point of the cord has this section been cut?
    A. Cervical
    B. Coccygeal
    C. Lumbar
    D. Sacral
    E. Thoracic

42. Which of the following make up the two main muscles of the pelvic floor?
    A. The coccygeus and transversus ani
    B. The levator ani and coccygeus
    C. The levator ani and internal oblique
    D. The obturator internus and external oblique
    E. The rectus abdominis and internal oblique

43. The extensors of the forearm attach distally to which bony structure?
    A. The acromion
    B. The coronoid process
    C. The distal third of the clavicle
    D. The lateral epicondyle
    E. The medial epicondyle

44. Which muscle of the pelvis is the most powerful hip flexor and a rotator of the thigh?
    A. Adductor longus
    B. Gluteus maximus
    C. Gracilis
    D. Iliopsoas
    E. Sartorius

45. The conducting zone of the respiratory tract involves all of the following, *except*:
    A. Bronchi
    B. Bronchioles

C. Respiratory bronchioles
D. Terminal bronchioles
E. Trachea

46. What percentage of corticospinal fibres pass down the anterior cortico-spinal tract?
A. 5%
B. 15%
C. 50%
D. 75%
E. 80%

47. Which of the following macroscopic grooves on the surface of the spinal cord is the most prominent?
A. Anterior lateral fissure
B. Anterior median fissure
C. Lateral fissure
D. Posterior lateral fissure
E. Posterior median fissure

48. Which one of the following is *not* an accurate statement regarding normal haemostasis in humans?
A. Primary haemostasis occurs as a result of exposed subendothelium.
B. Primary haemostasis involves platelet adhesion and aggregation.
C. Secondary haemostasis requires the activation of plasminogen.
D. The adhesion of platelets to damaged vascular endothelium is mediated by von Willebrand factor.
E. Tissue factor complexes with factor VII during clot initiation.

49. Which of the following lists corresponds correctly to the leukocytes in order from most abundant to least abundant?
A. Lymphocytes, neutrophils, monocytes, eosinophils, basophils
B. Monocytes, neutrophils, lymphocytes, basophils, eosinophils
C. Neutrophils, lymphocytes, basophils, monocytes, eosinophils
D. Neutrophils, lymphocytes, eosinophils, monocytes, basophils
E. Neutrophils, lymphocytes, monocytes, eosinophils, basophils

50. Which one of the following statements regarding plasma proteins is *not* true?
A. A reduction in plasma protein levels causes fluid to move into tissues.
B. Albumins are formed in the liver and are the least abundant plasma proteins.
C. Globulins are produced in the liver and by the immune system.
D. Plasma proteins are largely responsible for creating the osmotic pressure of blood.
E. Plasma proteins make up about 7% of the plasma.

Answers Paper 5

1. C – Endothelium
The three layers of a blood vessel, from innermost to outermost, are the intima, media and adventitia. The intima consists of the endothelium and subendothelial connective tissue. The endothelium is rich in chemical receptors, mediating systemic signals relating to blood vessel function. Just outside of the subendothelial layer is the elastica interna. The media is rich in smooth muscle cells, which regulate vascular tone.

2. B – B-lymphocytes give rise to plasma cells
B-lymphocytes (B-cells) give rise to plasma cells which produce antibodies (immunoglobulins). Most of the lymphocytes are found in the lymph nodes and spleen, with only a small proportion present in the bloodstream. T-lymphocytes (T-cells) act directly against virus-infected cells and tumour cells.

3. C – Classical pathway
In the classical complement pathway, C1 binds to the F_c portion of IgG or IgM antibody when bound to an antigen. The resulting complex is a C3 convertase, which cleaves C3 to C3b and C3a. The lectin pathway is similar to the classical pathway and is initiated by binding of mannose-binding lectin onto mannans (bacterial surfaces with polysaccharides containing mannose). The resulting complex again forms a C3 convertase.

4. B – Gastrocnemius
Gastrocnemius is a member of the superficial muscles of the posterior leg. Along with the soleus and the plantaris, the gastrocnemius inserts via the Achilles tendon. It facilitates both knee flexion and ankle plantar flexion. The gastrocnemius is supplied by the tibial nerve, a branch of the sciatic nerve.

5. B – 8
There are 8 pairs of cervical nerves, 12 pairs of thoracic nerves, 5 pairs of lumbar nerves, 5 pairs of sacral nerves and 1 pair of coccygeal nerves. While the number of pairs of spinal nerves generally mirrors the number of corresponding vertebrae, the cervical spine is an exception, with 8 pairs of nerves for 7 cervical vertebrae.

6. D – Expression of glycoprotein IIb/IIIa receptors
Platelet aggregation is thought to begin with an injury to a vessel wall exposing thrombogenic vessel wall collagen, to which platelets directly adhere.

Activation of adherent platelets leads to synthesis of a number of chemical mediators; crucial among these are arachidonic acid and thromboxane A2. Thromboxane A2 leads to platelet expression of GPIIb/IIIa receptors, the subsequent binding of fibrinogen and platelet aggregation.

7. B – β-Lactams
β-Lactams are a large group of antibiotics which range from the first discovered penicillin to the newer fourth-generation cephalosporins and carbapenems. The others listed have their own separate groups.

8. C – Vitamin B_{12} is indicated for the treatment of pernicious anaemia
Vitamin B_{12} is required for effective erythropoiesis and DNA synthesis. It can be administered intramuscularly and orally, and is indicated for the treatment of pernicious anaemia. Initial treatment requires regular weekly injections, but once serum vitamin B_{12} is normalized injections should be given at 3-monthly intervals.

9. A – Amlodipine
Amlodipine is a direct calcium channel blocker. Current British Hypertension Society and NICE guidelines suggest that either a calcium channel blocker or a thiazide diuretic is used as the first-line therapy for essential hypertension in individuals aged over 55, or in those of Afro-Caribbean origin of any age. Individuals aged under 55 should be initially treated with an ACE inhibitor.

10. C – Pulmonary artery
Deoxygenated blood is delivered to the right side of the heart by the superior and inferior vena cavae. On right ventricular contraction, deoxygenated blood is pumped into the lungs via the pulmonary artery. Oxygenated blood drains into the left atrium via the pulmonary veins, of which there are commonly four. Oxygenated blood is pumped from the left ventricle into systemic circulation via the aorta.

11. B – Aspirin inhibits platelet aggregation
Aspirin (acetylsalicylic acid) was originally derived from the willow tree. Children under the age of 12 are at risk of developing Reye syndrome with aspirin. Aspirin is an antiplatelet agent. Heparin, not aspirin, activates antithrombin III.

12. B – Left gastric vein
Oesophageal branches of the left gastric vein anastomose with oesophageal branches of the azygous system. In the context of portal hypertension, these anastomoses can form oesophageal varices, which in the event of rupture can cause a life-threatening upper GI bleed.

13. C – E-selectin
The word 'opsonization' derives from Greek *opsonein* – 'to prepare for the table'. In the same way, opsonization of bacteria makes them easier to target for phagocytosis. Collectins are a group of pattern

recognition receptors that bind to particular molecules on microbial surfaces and therefore act as opsonins independently of complement and antibodies. Mannose-binding lectin is an example of a collectin that recognizes carbohydrate units. Synergy between both antibody and complement provides stronger opsonization, but both can function independently. E-selectin is a receptor found on endothelial cells, which binds sialylated oligosaccharide on leukocytes to encourage margination of leukocytes during inflammation.

14. A – Hepatic vein
The inferior mesenteric vein joins first with the splenic vein, then the superior mesenteric vein, to form the portal vein. The portal vein supplies as much as 75% of the liver's blood supply (the remainder coming chiefly from the hepatic artery). The left gastric vein also drains into the portal vein but also anastomoses with the azygous system around the oesophagus. Blood leaves the liver via the hepatic vein and drains into the inferior vena cava. Obstruction of the hepatic vein can give rise to Budd–Chiari syndrome.

15. A – Arteriole
Vascular resistance is determined by the muscular vessels of the arterial side of the body's circulation. In particular, the smaller diameter arterioles are the chief determinant of vascular resistance.

16. E – Since the introduction of folic acid supplements for pregnant women, the rate of neural tube defects in newborn babies has fallen markedly
Folic acid is administered orally and has no contraindications or serious adverse effects. Folate is required for DNA synthesis and effective erythropoiesis. Folate deficiency can cause a macrocytic megaloblastic anaemia.

17. C – They compete with tRNA for the A-site
Tetracyclines are inhibitors of protein synthesis, where they specifically inhibit binding of aminoacyl-tRNA to the ribosome complex. Macrolides inhibit translocation. Aminoglycosides cause anticodon recognition which leads to the misreading of DNA. Chloramphenicol inhibits transpeptidation.

18. B – Fluoroquinolones
Ciprofloxacin is a fluoroquinolone. These antimicrobials inhibit topoisomerase II – a DNA gyrase – which consequently prevents the negative supercoiling of DNA.

19. D – Small amounts of iron are lost each day in urine and perspiration
Sixty-five percent of the body's iron supply is from haemoglobin. Iron is stored inside cells as ferritin and haemosiderin. The iron-transport protein in blood is transferrin, not ferritin. The average daily loss of iron is 1 mg, but this is higher in premenopausal women due to menstrual losses. Basal daily iron losses occur in urine and sweat.

20. B – Mycobacteria

The mechanism of action of ethambutol is unknown. However, it takes up to 24 hours before it begins to inhibit growth of mycobacteria. It cannot be used independently as resistance quickly develops.

21. C – Class III

Class III reactions represent the best targets as these involve the assembly of small molecules into macromolecules such as DNA and RNA. Class II represents the second best choice as these are the reactions which produce the small molecules such as amino acids. A drug which acts on this reaction is the group of sulphonamides. Class I reactions are an unhelpful target as there is no great difference between human and bacterial mechanisms. Classes IV and V do not exist.

22. D – Sulphonamides

Sulphonamides affect folate synthesis by inhibiting dihydropteroate synthetase. They are competitive inhibitors of the enzyme. While it produces dihydropteroate acid in bacteria, it has no function in humans. The others have no effect on folate synthesis.

23. C – It is caused by absent or faulty alpha or beta globin chains

Thalassaemias are typically seen in people of Mediterranean ancestry, such as Greeks and Italians. It is caused by absent or faulty alpha or beta globin chains. Thalassaemia is associated with an increased risk of infection. There are many subtypes of thalassaemia, but sickle cell disease is not one of them.

24. C – Clavulanic acid

Clavulanic acid has very little antimicrobial action on its own; however, by inhibiting β-lactamase, it allows other antibiotics to work against those pathogens which have developed a resistance to β-lactam antibiotics, for example co-amoxiclav.

25. B – C3b

Opsonization is a process by which microbes within the body can be highlighted for destruction by cells of the immune system. Complement C3b aids in the opsonization of microbes. The complement cascade is versatile in that different components are able to initiate different parts of the inflammatory response.

26. D – The renal arteries subdivide to form interlobar, arcuate and interlobular arteries

The kidneys are supplied by the paired renal arteries, which branch from the abdominal aorta directly below the superior mesenteric artery. The renal arteries subdivide into interlobar, arcuate and interlobular arteries. The afferent arterioles formed from the interlobular arteries supply the glomerular capillary bed, which sits inside Bowman's capsule, the site of filtration. The renal veins drain the kidneys into the inferior vena cava (IVC). Because the IVC lies to the right of the midline, the left renal vein is longer and receives the left suprarenal vein, the left gonadal vein and the left inferior phrenic vein, while the right renal vein enters the IVC directly without receiving further tributaries.

27. A – A membrane attack complex

The membrane attack complex is formed in five main steps by combining complement components C5b through C9 and acts by insertion of a pore through the cell membrane of its target. This pore then allows the efflux and influx of ions and small molecules, including water. Reactive oxygen species and hydrogen peroxide produce oxidative cell damage, which then triggers death by apoptosis. Elastase is an enzyme released from neutrophil granules causing destruction via digestion. Lipopolysaccharide, or endotoxin, is a molecule contained within the outer membrane of Gram-negative bacteria.

28. B – Fluoroquinolones

Ciprofloxacin is a fluoroquinolone. These antimicrobials inhibit topoisomerase II – a DNA gyrase – which consequently prevents the negative supercoiling of DNA.

29. A – C3a and C5a

Overactivation of the anaphylatoxins C3a and C5a can result in unwanted levels of hypotension in response to infection. C5a, in addition to acting to release histamine, is involved in leukocyte chemotaxis and activation. C3b binds glycoproteins on microbe cell surfaces and acts as an opsonin through specific binding to receptors on macrophages and neutrophils. C5b serves as an anchor for the formation of the membrane attack complex (MAC).

30. B – It is associated with neurological damage

Folic acid deficiency anaemia causes a form of megaloblastic anaemia identical to that seen in vitamin B_{12} deficiency but not associated with neurological damage. It may be due to dietary deficiency, e.g. in alcoholism and anorexia.

31. E – Reversible neurological damage

Vitamin B_{12} deficiency can lead to irreversible neurological damage. Pernicious anaemia is the most common form of vitamin B_{12} deficiency. It occurs more often in women than men, usually between 45 and 65 years of age.

32. B – Femoral head

Avascular necrosis (or osteonecrosis) is caused by an interruption of blood flow to the bone, resulting in necrosis of the cortex, medullary bone and marrow. The femoral head has limited collateral blood supply and so disturbance of its vasculature can result in ischaemia and subsequent necrosis. The patient may present with increasing hip pain and an inability to bear weight, followed by progressive limitation in the range of move-ment of the joint. Limb shortening occurs when bone destruction ensues. Predisposing factors to osteonecrosis include alcohol excess, corticoste-roid therapy, neck of femur fracture, dislocation, sickle cell disease and disseminated malignancy. It can also occur following scaphoid fractures.

33. A – Carbon dioxide complexes with haemoglobin to form carboxyhaemoglobin

Haemoglobin is contained in erythrocytes, rather than existing free in plasma. Carbon dioxide and haemoglobin combine to form carbamino-haemoglobin. Carbon monoxide readily combines with haemoglobin to form carboxyhaemoglobin. The other given statements are true.

34. D – Plasma proteins carry thyroid hormones

Water contributes to 90% of plasma volume. The plasma protein pool has the following composition: 60% albumin, 36% globulins, 4% fibrinogen. Steroid and thyroid hormones are carried by plasma proteins.

35. D – Na^+

Potassium is the primary cation of the intracellular fluid. Phosphates, calcium and magnesium are also found in higher concentrations intracel-lularly than extracellularly. Sodium ions are the most abundant cations of the extracellular fluid.

36. E – Stained basophils have U-shaped nuclei

Both basophils and mast cells bind to IgE. Eosinophils fight against para-sitic worms. Basophils are the least abundant white blood cell. It is their cytoplasm that contains histamine granules. Basophils stain purplish-black, and stained nuclei are generally U- or S-shaped with two or three conspicuous constrictions.

37. A – Membranous urethra

The male urethra is approximately 20 cm long and facilitates the pas-sage of urine and semen. It is divided anatomically into four sections: the intramural (preprostatic or vesicular), prostatic, intermediate (mem-branous) and spongy urethra. Most proximally, the preprostatic urethra runs vertically through the neck of the bladder. The prostatic urethra then passes vertically through the anterior prostate. The membranous, or intermediate, part of the urethra is the narrowest of the four parts and therefore the most vulnerable to trauma at instrumentation (e.g. catheter-ization). The most distal and longest part is the spongy (cavernous) ure-thra, which passes through the corpus spongiosum and ends in a slit-like opening (the external urethral meatus).

38. E – Vasopressin release is stimulated by an increase in plasma osmolality

Osmoreceptors within the anterior hypothalamus detect changes in plasma osmolality and secrete vasopressin (or antidiuretic hormone [ADH]) via the posterior pituitary gland in response to an increase in plasma osmolality. Oxytocin and vasopressin are synthesized within different neurons to allow independent release. A decrease in plasma volume, detected by the baroreceptors, will cause an increase in vasopressin release. Once activated by hypovolaemia, the increase in vasopressin is dramatic and may override signals from osmoreceptors in order to maintain plasma volume at the expense of decreasing osmolality.

39. A – Blood-borne erythropoietin stimulates the spleen to produce more erythrocytes

Erythropoietin is a naturally occurring hormone which is mainly produced by the liver and kidneys in response to hypoxic stress. This hormone stimulates the bone marrow to produce more red blood cells. The spleen is involved in the breakdown of old red blood cells.

40. A – Approximately two-thirds of total body water is intracellular

Water makes up a higher percentage of total body mass within males and infants (60% and 75%, respectively) than it does within females (roughly 50%). This is due to the relatively higher percentage of adipose tissue within women. Two-thirds of total body water (42 L) is contained within cells (intracellular). Of the remaining extracellular fluid, the majority is found within the interstitial spaces, and only 3 L of fluid is generally found within the intravascular plasma.

41. D – Sacral

The grey matter is largest in the sacral area, and at this point it occupies a significantly greater area in cross-section than the white matter. The grey matter contains neural cell bodies and is the major component of the central nervous system. The area of grey matter increases as the spinal cord descends.

42. B – The levator ani and coccygeus

The muscles of the pelvic floor consist of the levator ani and coccygeus. The levator ani is made up of four parts: levator prostatae/vaginae, puborectalis, pubococcygeus and iliococcygeus. The coccygeus is the posterior muscle of the pelvic floor. Levator ani can be damaged in pregnancy and childbirth. The pelvic floor muscles can be exercised and tone improved by Kegel exercises, which can help patients with stress incontinence and potentially protect against prolapse.

43. D – The lateral epicondyle

The lateral epicondyle is the attachment of the common extensor tendon of the forearm. Inflammation of the lateral epicondyle is known as 'tennis elbow', which results in tenderness over the lateral epicondyle and pain on wrist extension. It is common in activities that utilize repetitive wrist extension. The medial epicondyle is the common flexor origin, and inflammation occurring here is known as medial epicondylitis or 'golfer's elbow'.

44. D – Iliopsoas

The iliopsoas is made up of the iliacus and psoas major and facilitates hip flexion and external rotation. The sartorius muscle facilitates sitting cross-legged, while the gluteus maximus extends the hip along with the hamstring muscles. Both the adductor longus and gracilis are responsible for adduction and are supplied by the obturator nerve.

45. C – Respiratory bronchioles

The conducting zone of the respiratory tract, where convection of atmospheric gases takes place, includes the trachea, bronchi, bronchioles and terminal bronchioles. The transitional and respiratory zones, where diffusion of oxygen and carbon dioxide takes place, include respiratory bronchioles, alveolar ducts and alveolar sacs.

46. B – 15%

At the pyramidal decussation, 80% of corticospinal fibres pass into the contralateral lateral corticospinal tract. The remaining fibres remain uncrossed, with 15% passing into the ipsilateral anterior corticospinal tract and 5% descending in the ipsilateral lateral corticospinal tract.

47. B – Anterior median fissure

The anterior median fissure is the most prominent groove on the surface of the spinal cord. It is occupied by the anterior spinal artery. The posterior median fissure is less prominent and is only present in the medulla oblongata. The anterior and posterior nerve rootlets emerge at the anterior lateral and posterior lateral fissures. The lateral (Sylvian) fissure divides the frontal and temporal lobes from the parietal lobe.

48. C – Secondary haemostasis requires the activation of plasminogen

Plasminogen is necessary for the process of fibrinolysis to occur, i.e. for clot regulation and removal. Plasminogen is cleaved by tissue plasminogen activator (t-PA) to the fibrinolytic enzyme plasmin. All the other statements regarding haemostasis are correct.

49. E – Neutrophils, lymphocytes, monocytes, eosinophils, basophils

From most to least abundant, the leukocytes are: neutrophils, lymphocytes, monocytes, eosinophils and basophils. The following phrase may help you to remember the order: Never Let Monkeys Eat Bananas.

50. B – Albumins are formed in the liver and are the least abundant plasma proteins

Plasma proteins make up around 7% of the plasma and are largely responsible for creating the osmotic pressure of blood. If plasma protein levels fall, because of either reduced production or loss from the blood vessels, osmotic pressure is also reduced, and fluid moves into tissues (oedema) and body cavities. Albumins are the most abundant plasma proteins, comprising 60% of the total.

Questions Paper 6

1. What is the name of the four-carbon compound that is converted to oxaloacetate in the tricyclic acid cycle?
   A. Acetyl-CoA
   B. Citrate
   C. Oxaloacetate
   D. Oxoglutarate
   E. Succinate

2. Which one of the following statements regarding sickle cell disease is *least* accurate?
   A. Sickle cell disease produces shortened red blood cell survival.
   B. Sickle cell haemoglobin (HbS) results from a single base mutation, which produces a substitution of valine for thymine.
   C. Sickling may be precipitated by cold.
   D. The disease occurs mainly in people of African origin.
   E. The single base substitution of HbS occurs in the β-globin chain.

3. Which part of the small intestine contains the majority of the Brunner glands?
   A. Duodenum
   B. Ileum
   C. Jejunum
   D. All of the above
   E. None of the above

4. Which enzyme acts on oxaloacetate and acetyl-CoA in the citric acid cycle?
   A. Aconitase
   B. Citrate synthase
   C. Fumarate hydratase
   D. Isocitrate dehydrogenase
   E. Succinate dehydrogenase

5. Bone marrow can be found in which type of bone?
   A. Cancellous
   B. Compact
   C. Cortical
   D. Lamellar
   E. Woven

6. Citrate is a six-carbon compound found in the Krebs cycle. What other compound in the Krebs cycle contains six carbons?
   A. Fumarate
   B. Isocitrate
   C. Malate
   D. Oxoglutarate
   E. Succinate

7. Which one of the following is an opioid receptor?
   A. Gamma receptor
   B. Lambda receptor
   C. Mu receptor
   D. Omega receptor
   E. Sigma receptor

8. Which one of the following is a sesamoid bone?
   A. Femur
   B. Humerus
   C. Patella
   D. Scaphoid
   E. Tibia

9. In the citric acid cycle, succinyl-CoA is converted to succinate by which enzyme?
   A. Succinyl-CoA carboxylase
   B. Succinyl-CoA dehydrogenase
   C. Succinyl-CoA synthetase
   D. Succinyl dehydrogenase
   E. Succinyl synthetase

10. Which of the following is *not* a physiological effect of non-steroidal anti-inflammatory drug use?
    A. Analgesic
    B. Anti-inflammatory
    C. Antiplatelet
    D. Antipyretic
    E. Antispasmodic

11. Which one of the following is a selective cyclooxygenase-2 inhibitor?
    A. Aspirin
    B. Diclofenac
    C. Diflunisal
    D. Ibuprofen
    E. Rofecoxib

12. Which part of the small intestine contains the longest villi?
    A. Duodenum
    B. Ileum

C. Jejunum
D. All of the above
E. None of the above

13. What is formed during the conversion of succinyl-CoA to succinate in the Krebs cycle?
   A. ADP and HSCoA
   B. ATP and HSCoA
   C. GDP and HSCoA
   D. GMP and HSCoA
   E. GTP and HSCoA

14. Which one of the following statements regarding iron deficiency anaemia is most accurate?
   A. Around 10% of dietary iron is normally absorbed through the stomach.
   B. Blood film appearances include hyperchromic macrocytic cells.
   C. It is commonly caused by malabsorption in the Western world.
   D. Koilonychia is a recognized feature.
   E. Serum ferritin is raised.

15. Which one of the following statements is *not* accurate regarding platelets?
   A. The mean platelet diameter is 1–2 µm.
   B. The normal platelet count range for all ages is $150–250 \times 10^9$/L.
   C. Their normal lifespan is 7–10 days.
   D. They are produced predominantly by the bone marrow megakaryocytes.
   E. Storage granules within the platelet include dense granules.

16. Which one of the following statements about the left main bronchus is *incorrect*?
   A. It does not branch until entry into the hilum.
   B. It gives off two branches.
   C. It lies anterior to the descending aorta.
   D. It lies inferior to the pulmonary artery.
   E. It lies posterior to the oesophagus.

17. Which one of the following statements regarding blood cells is *not* true?
   A. All blood cells are derived from pluripotent stem cells.
   B. Blood islands are formed in the yolk sac in the third week of gestation.
   C. Red cells survive on average 120 days.
   D. The bone marrow becomes the main source of blood cells during normal childhood and adult life.
   E. The liver and the kidneys are the chief sites of haematopoiesis from 6 weeks to 7 months' gestation.

18. Which of the following is the most common cause of abdominal aneurysmal disease?
    A. Arteritis
    B. Connective tissue abnormality
    C. Cystic medial degeneration
    D. Infection
    E. Trauma

19. Which one of the following is true regarding the spleen?
    A. Blood enters the spleen via the splenic artery.
    B. It is situated in the right hypochondrium.
    C. It is the smallest lymphoid organ in the body.
    D. It is unnecessary to educate all patients about the risk of infection after splenectomy.
    E. Splenectomy is performed mainly for iron deficiency anaemia.

20. Which of the following is indicated as the first-line analgesic for a patient with migraine?
    A. Codeine
    B. Fentanyl
    C. Methysergide
    D. Morphine
    E. Paracetamol

21. A primary chronic inflammatory response can be triggered in various ways. Exposure to which one of the following would *not* result in a primary chronic inflammatory response?
    A. Asbestos fibres
    B. *Mycoplasma tuberculosis*
    C. Polio virus
    D. *Staphylococcus aureus*
    E. Urate crystals

22. What is suppuration?
    A. A blind ending tract communicating with an epithelial surface
    B. The accumulation of pus within a hollow viscus with a blocked outflow tract
    C. The formation of an abnormal communication between two epithelial surfaces
    D. The formation of cellular debris composed of living and dead neutrophils and bacteria
    E. The local accumulation of pus within a membrane

23. With respect to blood groups, which one of the following is true?
    A. The ABO blood group system involves naturally occurring IgG antibodies.
    B. The ABO system involves naturally occurring IgM anti-A and anti-B antibodies.

C. The blood groups are determined by antigens on the surface of all cells.
D. The major blood groups are Kell, Duffy and Kidd.
E. The rhesus blood group system involves naturally occurring IgM antibodies.

24. Which of the following is *not* a side-effect of paracetamol?
 A. Bradycardia
 B. Hypotension
 C. Leukopaenia
 D. Rash
 E. Thrombocytopaenia

25. The platelet count may rise significantly in each of the following conditions *except*:
 A. Bone marrow failure
 B. Hodgkin lymphoma
 C. Major surgery
 D. Splenectomy
 E. Ulcerative colitis

26. The adenomatous polyposis coli (*APC*) gene marks what for degradation?
 A. α-Cartenin
 B. α-Catenin
 C. β-Cartenin
 D. β-Catenin
 E. δ Cartenin

27. Which *one* of the following is true regarding haemophilia?
 A. Haemophilia A is also known as Christmas disease.
 B. Haemophilia A is associated with a prolonged bleeding time.
 C. Haemophilia A is inherited as an X-linked disorder.
 D. Haemophilia B is caused by a deficiency of factor VIII.
 E. Haemophilia is an acquired coagulation disorder.

28. Which one of the following types of bone is part of the appendicular skeleton?
 A. Pelvis
 B. Ribs
 C. Skull
 D. Sternum
 E. Vertebral column

29. Which one of the following cell types connects the periosteum to the bone?
 A. Merkel cells
 B. Remak bundles

C. Schwann cells
D. Sharpey fibres
E. None of the above

30. Within which layer is the Auerbach's plexus found?
    A. Lamina propria
    B. Muscularis externa
    C. Muscularis mucosa
    D. Serosa
    E. Submucosa

31. Which one of the following is a characteristic of bone?
    A. It contains mostly type II collagen.
    B. It has calcium phosphate as its major inorganic constituent.
    C. It is devoid of cells.
    D. It is mostly composed of water.
    E. It is strong due to its lamellar structure.

32. Which one of the following constitutes a combination of codeine and paracetamol?
    A. Co-codamol
    B. Co-dydramol
    C. Co-proxafol
    D. Co-tramadol
    E. Co-proxamol

33. Osteoid osteomas can arise from which tissue?
    A. Cortex
    B. Medullary cavity
    C. Periosteum
    D. All of the above
    E. None of the above

34. What are the spicules on spongy bone called?
    A. Canaliculi
    B. Lacunae
    C. Sharpey fibres
    D. Tomes process
    E. Trabeculae

35. Which one of the following is associated with withdrawal symptoms?
    A. Aspirin
    B. Diclofenac
    C. Hyoscine
    D. Morphine
    E. Paracetamol

36. A patient is recovering from a left hemicolectomy. In the immediate postoperative period, which of the following would be the most appropriate mechanism of analgesia?
   A. Epidural
   B. Non-steroidal anti-inflammatory drug
   C. Paracetamol
   D. Syringe driver
   E. Tramadol and morphine

37. Which of the following is an organic component of bone?
   A. Calcium phosphate
   B. Hydroxyapatite
   C. Type I collagen
   D. All of the above
   E. None of the above

38. Regarding Volkmann canals, which one of the following statements is true?
   A. They are almost exclusively found in cancellous bone.
   B. They are never found in compact bone.
   C. They run parallel to Haversian canals.
   D. They run perpendicular to Haversian canals.
   E. None of the above.

39. Which one of the following is a cardioselective beta-blocker?
   A. Mannitol
   B. Metoprolol
   C. Propranolol
   D. Sotalol
   E. Verapamil

40. Which one of the following is a contraindication to the use of paracetamol?
   A. Asthma
   B. Drug abuse
   C. Gastric ulcer
   D. Liver failure
   E. Uncontrolled bleeding

41. A 57-year-old man who had a non-ST elevation myocardial infarction 4 months ago subsequently had a stent inserted into his right coronary artery. He was initiated on aspirin, clopidogrel, ramipril, bisoprolol and atorvastatin. He is now having problems sustaining erections. Which drug is most likely responsible?
   A. Aspirin
   B. Atorvastatin

C. Bisoprolol
D. Clopidogrel
E. Ramipril

42. Pyrexia is a common clinical sign of acute inflammation. What physiological mechanism underlies this?
   A. Increased cellular activity and basal metabolic rate with a resultant release of heat
   B. Increased sympathetic stimulation causing increased sweating
   C. Increased TSH release from the pituitary gland increasing basal metabolic rate
   D. Resetting of the hypothalamic–pituitary axis to increase ACTH production
   E. Resetting of the hypothalamic thermostat by endogenous chemicals

43. Individuals with a mutated *p53* gene in their germ line have what increase in risk of developing cancer?
   A. 5 times increase
   B. 10 times increase
   C. 25 times increase
   D. 35 times increase
   E. 50 times increase

44. A 64-year-old man with severe community-acquired pneumonia is most at risk of developing which type of shock?
   A. Anaphylactic shock
   B. Cardiogenic shock
   C. Hypovolaemic shock
   D. Neurogenic shock
   E. Septic shock

45. Which of the following features is more commonly associated with acute, rather than chronic, inflammation?
   A. Fibrosis
   B. Granuloma formation
   C. Infiltration of macrophages
   D. Infiltration of neutrophils
   E. Production of interferon gamma

46. Which part of the small intestine contains the majority of the Peyer's patches?
   A. Duodenum
   B. Ileum
   C. Jejunum
   D. All of the above
   E. None of the above

47. Which one of the following mediators of inflammation is produced by the liver?
    A. Complement
    B. Nitric oxide
    C. Prostaglandin
    D. Serotonin
    E. Tissue necrosis factor

48. Which one of the following statements about the right main bronchus is *incorrect*?
    A. It descends more vertically than the left.
    B. It divides before entering the hilum.
    C. It gives off three branches.
    D. It is related anteriorly to the superior vena cava.
    E. It is related inferiorly to the azygous vein.

49. Which one of the following statements about bronchopulmonary segments is *incorrect*?
    A. Adjacent segments are communicating.
    B. Each lung has 10 bronchopulmonary segments.
    C. Each segment has its own neurovascular supply.
    D. Each segment is wedge-shaped.
    E. The right lung has three superior, two middle and five inferior discretely functioning segments.

50. Which part of the small intestine is lined with simple columnar epithelium?
    A. Duodenum
    B. Ileum
    C. Jejunum
    D. All of the above
    E. None of the above

Answers Paper 6

1. E – Succinate
Oxaloacetate is a four-carbon molecule. It reacts with a two-carbon molecule of acetyl-CoA to form the six-carbon compound citrate. At this point in the citric acid cycle, one molecule of carbon dioxide is removed to form a five-carbon compound called oxoglutarate. Another carbon dioxide molecule is removed to form the four-carbon compound succinate, which is converted via oxidation back into oxaloacetate so that it can be used again in another cycle of the citric acid cycle. The citric acid cycle is also known as the tricyclic acid cycle or the Krebs cycle.

2. B – Sickle cell haemoglobin (HbS) results from a single base mutation, which produces a substitution of valine for thymine
HbS results from a single base mutation of adenine to thymine, which produces a substitution of valine for glutamine at the sixth codon of the β-globin chain. All the other statements given are true.

3. A – Duodenum
Brunner glands are found in the submucosa of the duodenum. They are compound tubular glands found in the part of the duodenum proximal to the sphincter of Oddi. Their main function is to produce an alkaline secretion which protects the duodenum from acidic chyme (from the stomach) and which allows favourable conditions for intestinal enzymes.

4. B – Citrate synthase
Pyruvate is acted on by pyruvate dehydrogenase to form acetyl-CoA. Pyruvate can also be metabolized by pyruvate carboxylase to form oxaloacetate, which is an important intermediary in the TCA cycle. Acetyl-CoA is a two-carbon compound that binds with the four-carbon compound oxaloacetate, via the enzyme citrate synthase, to form the six-carbon compound citrate. Citrate is then acted on by the enzyme aconitase, which converts the citrate to an intermediate compound, *cis*-aconitate, by removing a water molecule. *cis*-Aconitate is further metabolized by the enzyme aconitase and is converted to isocitrate by adding a water molecule. Isocitrate is still a six-carbon compound but it has been structurally altered by the removal and addition of a water molecule. The six-carbon molecule of isocitrate is acted on by another enzyme, isocitrate dehydrogenase, to form the five-carbon compound, oxoglutarate. During the conversion of isocitrate to oxoglutarate, one molecule of NADH and one molecule of CO_2 are formed.

5. A – Cancellous
Cancellous bone (also known as spongy or trabecular bone) is where bone marrow tissue can be found. Compact (or cortical) bone is the harder outer layer of bone. The terms 'woven' and 'lamellar' refer to the way the bone is microscopically deposited: woven bone is disorganized and weaker, and it is gradually remodelled into the stronger and more organized lamellar type.

6. B – Isocitrate
Isocitrate is another six-carbon compound found in the Krebs cycle.

7. C – Mu receptor
Opioids are chemicals that bind to opioid receptors. There are three main opioid receptors, μ, κ and δ (mu, kappa and delta), although up to 17 have been described. They work principally on the μ receptor, which was so named after it was found to be responsible for morphine's action. There are three subtypes of μ-receptor: μ_1, μ_2 and μ_3. μ_1 receptors are associated with analgesia; μ_2 receptor activation results in respiratory depression and euphoria; and μ_3 receptors may result in vasodilation. Another important receptor is the opioid-receptor-like receptor 1 (ORL1), which is involved in pain responses and plays a role in the development of tolerance to μ-opioid agonists used as analgesics. All the opioid receptors are G-protein-coupled receptors that affect GABA neurotransmission. Common side-effects of opioids include nausea, vomiting, drowsiness, itching, dry mouth, respiratory depression, miosis (papillary constriction), dependence, tolerance, constipation and hallucinations.

Most adverse effects can be managed as follows:

- Nausea and vomiting – antiemetics such as metoclopramide or the 5-HT3 antagonist ondansetron
- Drowsiness – CNS stimulants such as caffeine
- Itching – antihistamines
- Respiratory depression – respiratory stimulants, e.g. doxapram
- Constipation – laxatives
- All opioid effects can be reversed using an opioid antagonist such as naloxone

8. C – Patella
A sesamoid bone is a bone which develops within a tendon or muscle. The largest example is the patella, which is found within the quadriceps tendon. Sesamoid bones are used to modify pressure, to diminish friction, and occasionally to alter the direction of a muscle pull.

9. C – Succinyl-CoA synthetase
Succinyl-CoA is metabolized by the enzyme succinyl-CoA synthetase to form succinate. During this process, a molecule of both guanosine triphosphate and HSCoA is formed. These are removed from the cycle.

10. E – Antispasmodic

NSAIDs inhibit cyclooxygenase (COX) enzymes. They are analgesics, anti-inflammatories, antipyretics and antiplatelets. They do not relieve bowel spasm.

11. E – Rofecoxib

Rofecoxib is a selective inhibitor of the isoenzyme cyclooxygenase COX-2. It is therefore thought not to have gastrointestinal side-effects, which occur secondary to COX-1 inhibition. However, long-term use of selective COX-2 inhibitors has been associated with an increased risk of cardiovascular thrombotic events, and these have therefore been withdrawn. It should be noted that non-selective NSAIDs have also been associated with a small increase in the risk of thrombotic events, and thus the lowest effective dose should always be prescribed for the shortest period of time possible.

12. C – Jejunum

The villi within the jejunum are much longer than those in the duodenum or ileum. They increase their area further with the presence of microvilli and consequently increase their nutrient absorption. They also have large circular folds within the submucosa which allow for an increase in the surface area. In comparison to more proximal parts of the small intestine, the ileal villi are far shorter. This is due to its main function of vitamin B_{12} and bile salt absorption, so less absorptive capacity is required.

13. E – GTP and HSCoA

During the conversion of succinyl-CoA to succinate, a molecule of guanosine triphosphate (GTP) is formed, as well as a molecule of HSCoA. These are removed from the cycle.

14. D – Koilonychia is a recognized feature

Blood loss is the dominant cause of iron deficiency in the Western world. Laboratory findings would show hypochromic, microcytic cells. Circulating serum ferritin and iron are reduced, alongside increased transferrin levels and unsaturated iron binding capacity. Iron is primarily absorbed through the duodenum. Characteristic (although relatively uncommon) features of iron deficiency include koilonychias (spoon-shaped nails), glossitis, pica (an appetite for non-nutritive substances) and hair thinning.

15. B – The normal platelet count range for all ages is 150–250 × 10⁹/L

The reference range for platelet levels in most hospital laboratories is between 150 and 400 × 10⁹/L. This reference range is applicable for all ages.

16. E – It lies posterior to the oesophagus

The left main bronchus gives off an upper and a lower lobe branch after entering the hilum. The left main bronchus lies anterior to both the oesophagus and descending aorta. The pulmonary artery lies above the left main bronchus.

17. E – The liver and the kidneys are the chief sites of haematopoiesis from 6 weeks to 7 months' gestation
Haematopoiesis (from the Greek *haema* = blood; *poiein* = to make) is the formation of blood cellular components. In developing embryos blood formation occurs in aggregates of blood cells in the yolk sac. As development progresses from 6 weeks, blood formation occurs in the spleen, liver and lymph nodes. In some vertebrates haematopoiesis occurs wherever there is a loose stroma of connective tissue, such as in the kidney or gut.

18. C – Cystic medial degeneration
Abdominal aneurysmal disease is a common and occasionally fatal condition. It is defined as a dilatation of the aorta of greater than 50% of its original diameter. Generally, it is a disease of old age. It is six times more common in men than women. The strongest aetiological factor is thought to be atherosclerosis, but there is also a strong familial component. Diabetes is thought to be protective. Cystic medial degeneration describes the loss of muscle and elastic fibres in the aortic media, and it is strongly associated with atherosclerosis and hypertension. The UK Small Aneurysm Trial has demonstrated that aneurysms can be safely monitored until they reach 5.5 cm in diameter size, become symptomatic or grow by more than 1 cm/year.

19. A – Blood enters the spleen via the splenic artery
The spleen is the largest lymphoid organ and is situated in the left hypochondrium. There is an increased risk of overwhelming infections in patients after splenectomy. Splenectomy is performed most frequently following traumatic injury.

20. E – Paracetamol
A patient with migraine should initially be treated with a simple analgesic, such as paracetamol. Morphine and codeine can exacerbate the nausea associated with migraine. Fentanyl is not indicated. Methysergide is used as migraine prophylaxis but is not effective in the acute setting.

21. D – *Staphylococcus aureus*
Inert materials such as crystals or synthetic fibres are unable to be eradicated, and so trigger a chronic inflammatory response. Viruses and certain bacteria (including *Mycoplasma tuberculosis*) also do this. Most staphylococcal infections will initiate an acute inflammatory response only. Giant macrophages form when multiple macrophage cell membranes fuse as they collectively try to engulf a material. This happens when they are faced with indigestible minerals (e.g. silica), or bacteria with indigestible cell walls (*M. tuberculosis*).

22. D – The formation of cellular debris composed of living and dead neutrophils and bacteria

Suppuration is the formation of cellular debris composed of living and dead neutrophils, bacteria and cellular debris (pus). The accumulation of pus within a membrane is called an abscess, and within a hollow viscus is an empyema. A fistula is an abnormal communication between two epithelial surfaces (apart from arteriovenous fistulae, which occur between two endothelial surfaces), and a sinus is a blind ending tract communicating with an epithelial surface.

23. B – The ABO system involves naturally occurring IgM anti-A and anti-B antibodies

The ABO blood group involved naturally occurring IgM antibodies, while rhesus (Rh) antibodies are usually IgG. The ABO and Rh systems are the two major blood group systems, although the Kell, Dufy and Kidd group systems are the next most clinically significant. Antigens on the surface of red cells only determine the blood groups.

24. A – Bradycardia

Bradycardia is not a documented side-effect of paracetamol use. Rashes, blood disorders and hypotension (when given intravenously) are rare side-effects of paracetamol.

25. A – Bone marrow failure

Bone marrow failure includes a group of disorders that can be either inherited or acquired. It can lead to an acutely or chronically impaired production of all or some of the blood cellular components.

26. D – β-Catenin

The *APC* gene marks β-catenin for degradation by ubiquitination. A deletion in the *APC* gene causes an increase in the cytoplasmic levels of β-catenin, which in turn leads to an increase in the nuclear levels of β-catenin, and this results in an increased transcription of genes associated with cellular proliferation.

27. C – Haemophilia A is inherited as an X-linked disorder

Haemophilia A (factor VIII deficiency) and haemophilia B (factor IX deficiency) are inherited coagulation disorders. Haemophilia A and B are inherited as an X-linked recessive disorder. Haemophilia B is also known as Christmas disease. Haemophilia A is associated with a normal bleeding time.

28. A – Pelvis

The appendicular skeleton describes the part of the skeleton that supports the limbs. It comprises the bones of the pectoral girdle, the pelvis and the upper and lower limbs. The axial skeleton comprises the bones of the skull, vertebral column, ribs and sternum. This is just one way of organizing the skeletal system.

29. E – None of the above
Sharpey fibres are composed of a matrix of connective tissue which connects the periosteum to the bone. Remak bundles are the eponymous name for groups of C-fibre axons. Schwann cells are a type of glial cell which cover an axon, and Merkel cells are found in the skin and are part of the somatosensory system.

30. B – Muscularis externa
Auerbach's plexus is part of the enteric nervous system. It is found between the longitudinal and circular layers of the muscularis externa. It provides both sympathetic and parasympathetic input to the gastrointestinal tract.

31. E – It is strong due to its lamellar structure
The mechanical properties of bone depend largely on its unique integrated lamellar structure. Hydroxyapatite is the primary mineral found in bone and the collagen is of type I.

32. A – Co-codamol
Co-codamol is a combination of codeine and paracetamol. Co-dydramol contains dihydrocodeine and paracetamol. Co-proxamol contains paracetamol and dextropropoxyphene. Neither co-tramadol nor co-proxafol exist.

33. D – All of the above
Osteoid osteomas are benign neoplasias which can arise from any of the periosteum, cortex or medullary cavity. Cortical tumours are the most common, accounting for up to 80% of all osteoid osteomas. They present with focal bone pain, which is often worse at night. Bone scans will show increased activity at the tumour site. They often regress spontaneously.

34. E – Trabeculae
Trabeculae are the spicules seen on spongy bones. They are the lattice-shaped network which forms the tissue. Canaliculi are the microscopic canals within the bone. An osteocyte rests in a space called a lacuna, which is situated between lamellae. Sharpey fibres are collagen fibres that extend into a bone at an angle. Tomes processes are extensions of odontoblast cells in the teeth that are involved in the production of enamel.

35. D – Morphine
Opioids are associated with dependence and both psychological and physiological withdrawal symptoms. Symptoms of opiate withdrawal include agitation, anxiety, muscle aches and sweating. Buprenorphine, a partial opioid receptor agonist, is a useful treatment of choice.

36. A – Epidural
An epidural is the most appropriate means of analgesia in this case, and this can be combined with a patient-controlled analgesia (PCA) system.

It provides adequate pain relief in the immediate stages postoperatively. Over the ensuing days, it can be weaned and replaced by intravenous analgesia.

37. C – Type I collagen
Type I collagen is the organic component of bone, whereas hydroxyapatite and calcium phosphate are inorganic components. These organic and inorganic components produce the matrix of the long bone. Type I collagen is also present in scar tissue, tendons and the endomysium of myofibrils.

38. D – They run perpendicular to Haversian canals
Volkmann canals – also known as perforating canals – are found in compact (cancellous) bone and run perpendicular to Haversian canals, connecting them with each other. The canals also carry small arteries which run throughout the bone.

39. B – Metoprolol
The cardioselective beta-blockers are atenolol, bisoprolol, metoprolol, nebivolol and acebutolol. These agents have a lesser effect on airway resistance compared to unselective beta antagonists. Under extreme caution and supervision, these drugs may be used in patients with a history of asthma or bronchoconstriction if there is no alternative (although this is a consultant decision). There is no clear long-term cardiovascular benefit of beta-blockers in uncomplicated hypertension.

40. D – Liver failure
An important but relative contraindication to the use of paracetamol is liver failure. Gastric ulceration, asthma and uncontrolled bleeding are contraindications to the use of non-steroidal anti-inflammatory drugs (NSAIDs).

41. C – Bisoprolol
Beta-blockers can have an adverse effect of impotence. It is extremely important to warn patients about this before starting them on this class of drugs, as they may be too embarrassed to present to their GP and end up living with a problem that is easily reversible. Beta-blockers can also cause nightmares, vivid dreams, hallucinations, poor effort tolerance and low mood, among many other side-effects.

42. E – Resetting of the hypothalamic thermostat by endogenous chemicals
Endogenous chemicals causing pyrexia are called pyrogens. Their release is stimulated by phagocytosis and by the presence of immune complexes and endotoxins (e.g. lipopolysaccharide). Examples of pyrogens include IL-2 and TNF. Their release results in increased levels of cyclooxygenase

and therefore prostaglandin production. In the hypothalamus, prosta-glandins, especially prostaglandin E2 (PGE2), stimulate neurotransmitters which reset the hypothalamic thermostat to a higher level. ACTH, pituitary hormones and the sympathetic system are not involved.

43. C – 25 times increase

People who have the p53 mutation in their germline have a 25 times increased risk of developing cancer. The *p53* gene is a tumour suppressor gene and is responsible for activating DNA repair in response to cell damage, inducing arrest of growth by halting the cell cycle at the G1/S phase and allowing any defects in DNA to be repaired at this stage, and in activating apoptosis in response to irreparable DNA damage.

44. E – Septic shock

Septic shock, like anaphylactic shock, is a form of distributive shock. Here, a systemic inflammatory reaction to an invading pathogen leads to a profound loss of vascular tone and a huge increase in capillary permeability. Subsequently there is insufficient peripheral resistance and cardiac preload to maintain an adequate blood pressure.

45. D – Infiltration of neutrophils

Neutrophils predominate within the acute phase of inflammation. Later, macrophages, lymphocytes and plasma cells predominate. Granulomas form in the presence of persistent T-cell activation, or in response to foreign material that cannot be digested. In both cases, the invading organism or substance is encircled by a wall of macrophages and lymphocytes (with or without fibroblasts and connective tissue). Fibrosis is the result of scar formation and collagen deposition and the tissue involved does not fully regain its structure or former function. Interferon gamma has antiviral actions and is produced by activated T-cells.

46. B – Ileum

Peyer's patches are organized lymphoid tissues which are nearly all found in the ileum in the small intestine. They appear to be oval or round in shape and are present in the lamina propria layer of the mucosa.

47. A – Complement

All the mediators given, apart from complement, are derived from cells within the location of inflammation. Nitric oxide is produced by endothelial cells, and prostaglandins by mast cells and leukocytes. Serotonin is a preformed mediator that is stored within platelet secretory granules, and TNF is produced by various cells including macrophages, endothelial cells and lymphocytes. Complement components are synthesized by the liver and travel to sites of inflammation whereupon they rely upon local activation.

48. D – It is related anteriorly to the superior vena cava

The azygous vein goes over the right main bronchus into the superior vena cava (SVC). The right main bronchus lies posterior to the SVC and ascending aorta. The right main bronchus descends more vertically than the left. It gives off three branches, one for each lobe of the right lung (upper, middle and inferior lobe branches). The right main bronchus gives off the branch for the upper lobe before entering the hilum.

49. A – Adjacent segments are communicating

Each lung has 10 wedge-shaped segments and each segment is a discretely functioning unit with its own neurovascular supply. There is no communication between the segments. As a result of the clear anatomical separation of these bronchopulmonary segments, a segment can be removed without influencing the function of neighbouring segments.

50. D – All of the above

The mucosa throughout the small intestine is lined with simple columnar epithelium. These cells are primarily enterocytes. They are often coated with a glycocalyx which contains digestive enzymes. On their apical surface there will be villi to increase the surface area. They are also able to secrete immunoglobulins.

Questions Paper 7

1. Which of the following benzodiazepines has the shortest duration of action?
   A. Diazepam
   B. Lorazepam
   C. Midazolam
   D. Nitrazepam
   E. Temazepam

2. Within which layer is the Meissner's plexus found?
   A. Lamina propria
   B. Muscularis externa
   C. Muscularis mucosa
   D. Serosa
   E. Submucosa

3. Which of the following statements best describes the action of parathyroid hormone (PTH) on the kidney?
   A. PTH decreases calcium reabsorption in the thick ascending limb of the Loop of Henle.
   B. PTH increases calcium reabsorption at the distal tubule.
   C. PTH increases glomerular filtration rate.
   D. PTH increases secretion of calcium by the renal tubules.
   E. PTH increases urinary excretion of calcium.

4. During periods of starvation, muscle proteins are broken down to supply the body with an energy source. Which one of the following statements regarding this biochemical pathway is correct?
   A. Gluconeogenesis is catalysed by glucagon in the liver.
   B. Muscle breakdown provides the liver with glycogen from which to form glucose.
   C. Muscle breakdown results in the release of glucose directly into the bloodstream.
   D. Muscle breakdown supplies the liver with pyruvate for gluconeogenesis.
   E. The liver converts fatty acids into glucose in response to muscle breakdown during periods of starvation.

5. Which one of the following statements is true regarding sympathetic innervation to the heart?
   A. Decreases the rate and force of contraction
   B. Increases the force of contraction and decreases the heart rate
   C. Increases the heart rate and decreases the force of contraction
   D. Increases the rate and force of contraction
   E. None of the above

6. Which of the following receptors, when bound to an appropriate ligand, would *not* induce activation of a phagocyte?
   A. CD4 receptor
   B. Clq receptor
   C. CR1 receptor
   D. Fc receptor
   E. Toll-like receptor

7. Which one of the following is the second messenger system involved in increasing heart rate and force of contraction?
   A. Calcium
   B. Cyclic adenosine monophosphate
   C. Cyclic guanosine monophosphate
   D. Inositol trisphosphate
   E. Nitric oxide

8. Which of the following is a life-threatening type of cellulitis which occurs in the submandibular space?
   A. Boerhaave syndrome
   B. Caplan syndrome
   C. Ludwig angina
   D. Ondine curse
   E. Prinzmetal angina

9. Acetylcholine slows the heart by acting on which one of the following receptors?
   A. Adrenergic receptors
   B. GABA receptors
   C. Glutamate receptors
   D. Muscarinic receptors
   E. None of the above

10. Which of the statements below regarding the erythrocyte sedimentation rate (ESR) is most likely to be correct?
   A. A low ESR occurs in infection.
   B. A low ESR occurs in malignancy.
   C. ESR is largely determined by plasma concentrations of white blood cells in the body.

D. ESR measures the rate of fall of a column of suspended red cells in 24 hours.

E. The normal range of ESR rises with increasing age.

11. Acetylcholine decreases the force of contraction of the heart by decreasing which one of the following?
   A. Calcium
   B. Cyclic guanosine monophosphate
   C. Inositol trisphosphate
   D. Intracellular cyclic adenosine monophosphate
   E. Nitric oxide

12. Which of the following is most likely to be seen in acute epiglottitis?
   A. Cervical adenopathy
   B. Tender larynx
   C. Tonsillar enlargement
   D. Tonsillar exudate
   E. Trismus

13. Activation of the parasympathetic postganglionic neurons innervating the bladder wall results in which of the following?
   A. Contracts and relaxes the smooth muscle
   B. Contracts the smooth muscle
   C. Relaxes the smooth muscle
   D. Both (A) and (B)
   E. None of the above

14. In relation to the bladder, postganglionic fibres from sympathetic neurons pass via which nerve?
   A. Common peroneal nerve
   B. Genital branch of the genitofemoral nerve
   C. Hypogastric nerve
   D. Ilioinguinal nerve
   E. Sciatic nerve

15. Erectile tissue is controlled by which of the following?
   A. Both parasympathetic and sympathetic systems
   B. Parasympathetic system and the release of acetylcholine
   C. Parasympathetic system and the release of nitric oxide
   D. Sympathetic system and the release of adrenaline
   E. Sympathetic system and the release of nitric oxide

16. Which one of the following best describes the correct structure of the platelet?
   A. Aspirin promotes the formation of new platelets.
   B. Platelets are anucleate.
   C. Platelets are cells and therefore contain nuclei.

D. Platelets survive for longer than 120 days.

E. Their biconcave shape enhances oxygen delivery at the cellular level.

17. Which one of the following conditions and modes of inheritance match correctly?
    A. Haemophilia A: autosomal recessive
    B. Haemophilia B: autosomal recessive
    C. Hereditary spherocytosis: autosomal dominant
    D. Sickle cell disease: autosomal dominant
    E. Thalassaemia: sex-linked

18. A 29-year-old woman presents to her GP with weight loss and palpitations. Examination reveals a diffuse smooth neck swelling. Which one of the following medications should be commenced?
    A. Carbimazole
    B. Digoxin
    C. Hydrocortisone
    D. Levothyroxine
    E. Liothyronine

19. Benzodiazepines act through which of the following mechanisms?
    A. 5-HT receptor agonism
    B. Beta adrenoceptor antagonism
    C. GABA receptor agonism
    D. Serotonin agonism
    E. None of the above

20. The axon from preganglionic neurons of the autonomic nervous system is:
    A. Myelinated and its cell body is found in the autonomic ganglion
    B. Myelinated and its cell body is found in the central nervous system
    C. Myelinated and its cell body is found in the peripheral nervous system
    D. Unmyelinated and its cell body is found in the central nervous system
    E. Unmyelinated and its cell body is found in the peripheral nervous system

21. A woman is due to have an elective subtotal thyroidectomy. Carbimazole was stopped 14 days previously. Which one of the following medications should be commenced preoperatively?
    A. Levothyroxine
    B. Liothyronine
    C. Potassium iodide
    D. Propranolol
    E. Propylthiouracil

22. A 32-year-old man presents to the emergency department with a 1-week history of lethargy and fever. Examination reveals a pulse rate of 96 beats/minute and a mildly enlarged thyroid gland with tenderness

to palpation. Thyroid function tests show mild hyperthyroidism and there was a low thyroid uptake on scintiscan. What is the ideal treatment in this scenario?

A. Carbimazole
B. Ibuprofen
C. Levothyroxine
D. Liothyronine
E. Propranolol

23. Which one of the following is true about tetracyclines?
A. They are associated with very few side-effects.
B. They are bactericidal.
C. They are bacteriostatic.
D. They inhibit DNA gyrase.
E. They inhibit transpeptidation.

24. Which of the following is the main active metabolite of diazepam?
A. Desmethylflurazepam
B. Nordazepam
C. Triazolam
D. Zolpidem
E. None of the above

25. What is the danger of selective cyclooxygenase 2 enzyme inhibition?
A. Increased risk of gastric ulceration.
B. Inhibition of prostacyclin production is greater than inhibition of thromboxane A2 production.
C. Inhibition of thromboxane A2 production is greater than prostacyclin production.
D. Leukotriene production is uninhibited.
E. Negligible danger.

26. Three days post-total thyroidectomy, a patient exhibits symptoms of numbness around her lips and tingling in her fingers. Examination reveals a positive Chvostek sign. Treatment with which one of the following should be commenced?
A. Calcium gluconate
B. Carbimazole
C. Levothyroxine
D. Pamidronate
E. No treatment required

27. Which one of the following is an antagonist of histamine and noradrenaline receptors?
A. Clozapine
B. Olanzapine
C. Quetiapine

D. Risperidone
E. Sertindole

28. The parasympathetic system forms part of which of the following?
   A. Autonomic nervous system
   B. Central nervous system
   C. Peripheral nervous system
   D. All of the above
   E. None of the above

29. The autonomic nervous system motor pathways typically consist of how many neurones?
   A. One
   B. Two
   C. Three
   D. Four
   E. Six

30. The axon from postganglionic neurons of the autonomic nervous system is:
   A. Myelinated and its cell body is found in the autonomic ganglion
   B. Myelinated and its cell body is found in the central nervous system
   C. Unmyelinated and its cell body is found in the autonomic ganglion
   D. Unmyelinated and its cell body is found in the central nervous system
   E. Unmyelinated and its cell body is found in the peripheral nervous system

31. Which one of the following drugs is associated with a risk of agranulocytosis?
   A. Clozapine
   B. Haloperidol
   C. Olanzapine
   D. Quetiapine
   E. Risperidone

32. In chemotaxis, the binding of chemotaxins to leukocyte G-protein cell receptors causes an increase in which of the following?
   A. Adenosine triphosphate (ATP) and basal metabolic activity
   B. Cytosolic calcium and contraction of microtubules
   C. Cytosolic calcium and growth of pseudopods
   D. Formation of mRNA and growth of flagella
   E. Formation of nucleic acids and enlargement of cell nucleus

33. Which one of the following is a D_2/D_3 receptor antagonist?
   A. Amisulpride
   B. Clozapine
   C. Olanzapine
   D. Quetiapine
   E. Risperidone

34. Preganglionic neurons of the parasympathetic division are situated in four cranial nerve nuclei in the brain stem. These are:
    A. Glossopharyngeal, vagus, optic and abducens
    B. Oculomotor, facial, glossopharyngeal and vagus
    C. Oculomotor, vagus, trochlear and trigeminal
    D. Olfactory, hypoglossal, accessory and vagus
    E. Optic nerve, oculomotor, trigeminal and facial nerve

35. Adhesion of leukocytes to endothelial cells is mediated by which type of receptor expressed on leukocyte cell surfaces?
    A. E-selectin
    B. Integrins
    C. Intercellular adhesion molecule 1
    D. L-selectin
    E. P-selectin

36. Once within the interstitium, leukocytes migrate towards the site of injury by chemotaxis. Which of the following molecules would *not* induce leukocyte chemotaxis?
    A. C5a
    B. Chemokines
    C. IgG
    D. Leukotriene B4
    E. Platelet activating factor

37. In the parasympathetic system, preganglionic neurons originating from nuclei of cranial nerve III synapse where?
    A. Ciliary ganglion
    B. Coeliac ganglion
    C. Inferior mesenteric ganglion
    D. Submandibular ganglion
    E. Superior mesenteric ganglion

38. Which one of the following statements concerning lung development is *incorrect*?
    A. A tracheal bud forms from the foregut.
    B. Alveolar development continues until 2 years of age.
    C. At 16 weeks' gestation, bronchial branching is complete.
    D. Different tissues within the lung develop at different rates.
    E. Malformation of the lung is dependent on the timing of the insult rather than the nature of the insult.

39. Which one of the following definitions best describes phagocytosis?
    A. Cellular death initiated from within the cell itself
    B. Excretion of substances within cell vesicles by fusion with the cell membrane
    C. Regrowth of blood vessels following injury

D. The engulfment and digestion of solid particles by cells

E. The intake of fluid into a cell by engulfment

40. Which one of the following statements about alveoli is *incorrect*?
    A. Alveoli account for the greatest proportion of lung volume.
    B. Gas exchange occurs through the alveolar basement membrane.
    C. Type I alveolar cells are thick cells providing structural integrity to the surface lining.
    D. Type I alveolar cells make up 90% of the alveolar surface lining.
    E. Type II alveolar cells produce surfactant.

41. In the parasympathetic system, preganglionic neurons originating from cranial nerve VII nuclei synapse where?
    A. Ciliary ganglion
    B. Coeliac ganglion
    C. Otic ganglion
    D. Pterygopalatine ganglion
    E. Superior cervical ganglion

42. Stimulation of secretion of the lacrimal and salivary glands is mediated via which of the following cranial nerves?
    A. Cranial nerve II
    B. Cranial nerves VII/IX
    C. Cranial nerve X
    D. Cranial nerve XI
    E. Cranial nerve XII

43. Which one of the following is *not* a common symptom of acute epiglottitis?
    A. Cough
    B. Drooling
    C. Dysphagia
    D. Fever
    E. Stridor

44. In the upper gastrointestinal tract, parasympathetic innervation:
    A. Decreases secretions, peristalsis and contraction of sphincters
    B. Decreases secretions, peristalsis and relaxation of sphincters
    C. Increases secretions, decreases peristalsis and relaxation of sphincters
    D. Increases secretions, peristalsis and contraction of sphincter
    E. Increases secretions, peristalsis and relaxation of sphincter

45. Which eicosanoid stimulates chemotaxis of neutrophils?
    A. Leukotriene B4
    B. Leukotriene C4
    C. Prostacyclin PGI2
    D. Prostaglandin PGE2
    E. Thromboxane A2

46. A patient suffering with a quinsy may have what pathognomonic symptom?
    A. Barking voice
    B. Hot potato voice
    C. Quack cough
    D. Rose spots
    E. None of the above

47. Which eicosanoid increases the sensitivity of pain receptors and can aid the production of fever?
    A. Leukotriene B4
    B. Leukotriene C4
    C. Prostacyclin PGI2
    D. Prostaglandin PGE2
    E. Thromboxane A2

48. Why does regular ingestion of aspirin or ibuprofen result in an increased risk of gastric ulcer formation?
    A. Inhibition of cyclooxygenase 1 (COX-1)
    B. Inhibition of lipoxygenase
    C. Inhibition of phospholipase A2
    D. Selective inhibition of cyclooxygenase 2 (COX-2)
    E. Stimulation of hydrogen ion release

49. During peristalsis, the activation of enteric neurons occurs via which one of the following receptors?
    A. Adrenergic receptors
    B. GABA receptors
    C. Glutamate receptors
    D. Muscarinic receptors
    E. Nicotinic receptors

50. Select the option below that correctly displays the order of events by which neutrophils locate an active area of inflammation

    A. Adhesion of integrins to endothelium, margination and rolling, diapedesis and phagocytosis of microbials
    B. Chemotaxis towards site of injury, margination and rolling, adhesion of integrins to endothelium and diapedesis
    C. Chemotaxis towards site of injury, margination and rolling, adhesion of integrins to endothelium, phagocytosis of microbials
    D. Diapedesis, adhesion of integrins to endothelium, margination and rolling, chemotaxis towards site of injury
    E. Margination and rolling, adhesion of integrins to endothelium, diapedesis, chemotaxis towards site of injury

Answers Paper 7

1. C – Midazolam

Midazolam is an ultra-short-acting benzodiazepine with a half-life of 2 hours and duration of action of less than 6 hours, making it an ideal premedication for surgery. This is compared to diazepam which has a long duration of action, up to 100 hours, because diazepam first metabolizes to the metabolically active desmethyldiazepam, oxazepam and temazepam.

2. C – Muscularis mucosa

Meissner's plexus (submucosal plexus) innervates the small intestine with parasympathetic fibres and is found in the muscularis mucosa. The nerve bundles within the submucosal plexus innervate the cells within the epithelial layer and the smooth muscle of the muscularis mucosa.

3. B – PTH increases calcium reabsorption at the distal tubule

Parathyroid hormone (PTH) is released by the parathyroid glands in response to low extracellular calcium. In order to normalize plasma calcium, PTH acts on bone to increase osteoclastic activity and bone demineralization, which results in the release of calcium. PTH also stimulates the conversion of vitamin D to its active form, 1,25-dihydroxycholecalciferol, which increases intestinal absorption of calcium. Finally, PTH increases the reabsorption of filtered calcium at both the thick ascending limb of the Loop of Henle and the distal tubule, thus conserving calcium by reducing its urinary excretion.

4. D – Muscle breakdown supplies the liver with pyruvate for gluconeogenesis

During periods of starvation, muscle proteins can be utilized for gluconeogenesis. By definition, gluconeogenesis is the formation of glucose from non-carbohydrate precursors. Amino acids (mainly alanine) from muscle proteins provide the source of pyruvate for gluconeogenesis in the liver:

$$2\,\text{Pyruvate} + 2\,\text{NADH} + 4\,\text{ATP} + 2\,\text{GTP} + 4H_2O$$
$$\rightarrow \text{Glucose} + 2\,\text{NAD}^+ + 4\,\text{ADP} + 2\,\text{GDP} + 2\,H^+ + 6\,P_i$$

Alcohol reduces the ability of the liver to perform gluconeogenesis. Ethanol creates high levels of NADH, which promotes the formation of lactate from pyruvate, thus reducing the amount of pyruvate available for gluconeogenesis.

5. D – Increases the rate and force of contraction
The sympathetic division of the autonomic nervous system exhibits a flight-or-fight response, thus increasing both the heart rate and the force of contraction.

6. A – CD4 receptor
Toll-like receptors (TLRs) are a family of pattern recognition receptors within macrophages, mast cells and dendritic cells. TLRs detect the presence of invading microorganisms by identifying common molecules within their membranes. Lipopolysaccharide, for example, is the main ligand for TLR-4. Binding of a ligand induces an inflammatory and innate immune response. The Fc receptor (contained, for example, within macrophage and neutrophil membranes) binds specifically to the Fc region of an antibody. The Clq receptor recognizes the first component of the complement pathway. CR1 receptors bind to C3b. Both antibodies and complement components act as opsonins to induce phagocytosis and superoxide production. CD4 is a co-receptor for MHC class II molecules, expressed by T-lymphocytes during recognition of a foreign antigen.

7. B – Cyclic adenosine monophosphate
The signalling conduction pathway involved in increasing the rate and force of contraction of the heart is mediated via the cAMP (cyclic adenosine monophosphate) second messenger system. Normally, chemical transmitters that reach a receptor situated in the plasma membrane activate transducer proteins such as the G protein. This in turn activates the primary key effector enzymes, which generate a second messenger activating a secondary effector or acting directly on the target organ. The cAMP second messenger is produced by adenylyl cyclase following its activation by a G protein, while the primary effector enzyme that activates the inositol polyphosphate pathway is protein kinase C.

8. C – Ludwig angina
Ludwig angina is a rare but life-threatening infection most often caused by *Streptococcus*. The word 'angina' is derived from the Greek *ankhone* = strangling. Ludwig angina is an infection of the tissues in the floor of the mouth, often with concomitant dental infection.

9. D – Muscarinic receptors
Muscarinic receptors are present in the cardiocytes of the sinoatrial and atrioventricular nodes of the heart. The effect of acetylcholine on the muscarinic receptors of these nodes is to increase the resting K^+ conductance, resulting in a decrease in heart rate.

10. E – The normal range of ESR rises with increasing age
ESR measures the rate of fall of a column of red cells in plasma in 1 hour. It is largely determined by the plasma concentrations of proteins, especially fibrinogen and globulins. The normal range for ESR rises with age.

A raised ESR occurs in inflammatory disorders, infections, malignancy, myeloma, anaemia and pregnancy.

11. D – Intracellular cyclic adenosine monophosphate
The release of acetylcholine from parasympathetic nerve terminals, which then acts on muscarinic receptors in the cardiocytes of the cardiac muscle, leads to an increase in the resting K^+ conductance in these cells. This rise in K^+ conductance hyperpolarizes the cell, therefore reducing the rate of contraction. The decrease in force of contraction is mediated by down-regulating intracellular cAMP and subsequently reducing the L-type Ca^{2+} channels that are responsible for excitation–contraction.

12. B – Tender larynx
Acute epiglottitis is the result of localized *Haemophilus influenzae* infection of the supraglottic larynx. It is a medical emergency as the inflamed epiglottis can cause complete airway obstruction. Do not lay the patient down; keep them upright and as calm as possible. Immediate assessment by ENT and anaesthetics is required. Note that following the introduction of the Hib (*Haemophilus influenza* type B) vaccine the incidence of epiglottitis has reduced.

13. B – Contracts the smooth muscle
Parasympathetic innervation causes contraction and encourages emptying of the bladder. Postganglionic neurons in the pelvic ganglion mediate contraction of the bladder's smooth muscle.

14. C – Hypogastric nerve
Postganglionic fibres from sympathetic neurons innervate the bladder through the hypogastric nerve. When the sympathetic system is activated, the parasympathetic system is inhibited leading to relaxation of the bladder smooth muscle and contraction of the internal sphincter.

15. C – Parasympathetic system and the release of nitric oxide
The parasympathetic system is largely responsible for the erection. Parasympathetic innervation leads to the release of neurotransmitters and local mediators, including nitric oxide, which relaxes the vascular smooth muscle in the penis. There is dilation of the penis and blood fills the blood sinuses, resulting in an increase in the size of the erectile tissues. This causes compression of the superficial veins (which normally drain the penis), leading to engorgement and rigidity.

16. B – Platelets are anucleate
Platelets do not have nuclei. Platelets do not survive longer than 7 days and are inhibited by aspirin. Red blood cells are biconcave in shape, which provides a large surface area for oxygen transfer and therefore delivery at a cellular level.

17. C – Hereditary spherocytosis: Autosomal dominant
Hereditary spherocytosis is a genetically linked autosomal dominant form of spherocytosis. It is a genetic disorder of the red blood cell membrane and

can cause anaemia, jaundice and splenomegaly. Both haemophilia A and B are sex-linked genetic disorders. Both thalassaemia and sickle cell disease are autosomal recessive disorders.

18. A – Carbimazole
This woman has hyperthyroidism most likely due to Graves disease. This is an autoimmune condition resulting from IgG antibodies mimicking thyroid-stimulating hormone (TSH) and binding to TSH receptors on the thyroid gland, thus initiating production of thyroid hormones. This produces symptoms of hyperthyroidism and therefore carbimazole would be the drug of choice to control this condition.

19. C – GABA receptor agonism
Benzodiazepines act as $GABA_A$ receptor stimulators. Enhancing the effects of $GABA_A$ results in sedation, hypnosis and anxiolysis.

20. B – Myelinated and its cell body found in the central nervous system
The axon of a preganglionic neuron is a small-diameter, myelinated type B fibre extending to autonomic ganglion, and therefore transmits motor impulses from the central nervous system to autonomic ganglia.

21. C – Potassium iodide
Potassium iodide is used in optimizing hyperthyroid patients for surgery. This is due to its effect of inhibiting iodination of thyroglobulin, thus reducing thyroid hormone synthesis. Eventually the thyroid gland reduces in size and vascularity and therefore it is a useful medication to give prior to thyroidectomy.

22. B – Ibuprofen
This patient shows signs and symptoms of de Quervain thyroiditis. This is normally caused by a viral infection, producing symptoms typical of a viral illness and inflammatory changes in the thyroid gland causing tenderness and enlargement. The inflammatory damage can occasionally result in a transiently increased thyroid hormone secretion. The condition is usually self-limiting but non-steroidal anti-inflammatory drugs may be used for symptomatic relief.

23. C – They are bacteriostatic
Tetracyclines are bacteriostatic, which means they act to inhibit the growth of a bacterium which gives the body time to mount the appropriate defence.

24. B – Nordazepam
Nordazepam (N-desmethyldiazepam) is the active metabolite of diazepam and has a half-life of 60 hours. This leads to the lengthy metabolic activity of diazepam.

25. B – Inhibition of prostacyclin production is greater than inhibition of thromboxane A2 production

Selective COX-2 inhibition is associated with an increased production of thromboxane A2 (which causes vasoconstriction and indirect activation of platelet aggregation) out of proportion to prostacyclin (a vasoconstrictor). This results in an increased risk of thrombosis.

26. A – Calcium gluconate

Hypocalcaemia is a complication of post-thyroid surgery due to inadvertent damage or removal of the parathyroid glands. Serum calcium levels should be measured, and the patient should be observed for symptoms of hypocalcaemia in the first few days postoperatively (i.e. numbness and tingling of the hands/feet/lips, light-headedness and muscle weakness and cramps). In severe symptomatic hypocalcaemia, intravenous calcium gluconate must be immediately commenced. Mild asymptomatic hypocalcaemia can be treated with oral calcium and vitamin D supplementation. Chvostek sign – twitching of facial muscles after stimulation of the facial nerve by tapping over the masseter muscle at the angle of the jaw – is observed in hypocalcaemia.

27. D – Risperidone

Risperidone, as well as acting as a serotonin–dopamine atypical antipsychotic, is an antagonist of histamine and noradrenaline receptors. It is also known to cause the highest rise in prolactin of the antipsychotics.

28. B – Central nervous system

The nervous system consists of three parts: peripheral, central and autonomic. The autonomic nervous system consists of the nerve cells found within the sympathetic and parasympathetic nervous systems. It is mainly concerned with the innervation and regulation of visceral organs, smooth muscle and secretory glands.

29. B – Two

The autonomic nervous system efferent neurons differ from those of the somatic nervous system because of the two neurons between the central nervous system and the target organ. The first neuron is referred to as the preganglionic neuron and the second is the postganglionic neuron.

30. C – Unmyelinated and its cell body is found in the autonomic ganglion

The axon of a preganglionic neuron is a small-diameter, myelinated type B fibre extending to autonomic ganglion, and therefore transmits motor impulses from the central nervous system to autonomic ganglia.

31. A – Clozapine

Clozapine is known to cause agranulocytosis in 1% of patients. Consequently, patients will need to have their white cell count monitored regularly. The usual testing regimen is once every week for 6 months, every 2 weeks for the next 6 months and monthly thereafter (assuming agranulocytosis does not develop during this time).

32. B – Cytosolic calcium and contraction of microtubules

G-protein receptors are transmembrane receptors and therefore have a surface in contact with both the inside and outside of a cell. Chemotaxin binding to a receptor on the external surface of the cell results in activation of a G-protein on the inside surface. G-protein activation results in a cascade of reactions. Within leukocytes, this leads to the release of calcium within the cell cytoplasm. Calcium is required for the contraction of microtubules via actin and myosin filaments. When co-ordinated, this produces movement of the leukocyte towards the chemotaxin. This process is called chemotaxis.

33. A – Amisulpride

Amisulpride is an atypical antipsychotic which is a dopamine D_2/D_3 receptor antagonist and is used to treat the positive symptoms of psychosis. Quetiapine acts on D_{1-4} receptors. Olanzapine acts on D_2 receptors alone.

34. B – Oculomotor, facial, glossopharyngeal and vagus

The oculomotor, facial, glossopharyngeal and vagus nerves have axons that originate from preganglionic neurons which synapse at their respective terminal ganglia. Oculomotor preganglionic parasympathetic neurons originate from the Edinger–Westphal nucleus and end in the ciliary ganglion. Postganglionic neurons travel in short ciliary nerves to supply the sphincter pupillae muscle of the iris and ciliary muscles, which play a key role in pupillary constriction in the pupillary light reflex. In order to regulate the amount of light entering the eye, the size of the pupil serves as a controlled gateway. The illumination of the retina leads to the pupil constriction via contraction of the sphincter pupillae muscle of the iris, thereby modulating the amount of light reaching the retina. This is known as the direct reflex. The indirect reflex is when the constriction of the pupil of the non-illuminated eye takes place without direct illumination of the retina – also known as the consensual light reflex. Facial preganglionic parasympathetic neurons originate from the superior salivatory nucleus of the pons (second part of the brain stem) and exit the brain stem in the sensory root of the facial nerve, also known as nervus intermedius. From here they travel via their terminal ganglia (submandibular and pterygopalatine) en route to innervating the submandibular and sublingual salivary glands, lacrimal gland, and nasal and oral mucous membranes. Glossopharyngeal parasympathetic neurons originate from the inferior salivatory nucleus of the medulla (third part of the brain stem), which subsequently synapse with postganglionic neurons in the otic ganglion which essentially innervates the parotid salivary gland.

Vagal parasympathetic neurons originate from the dorsal motor nucleus of the vagus, which is situated in the medulla underneath the floor of the fourth ventricle. From here they travel to the cardiovascular, respiratory and gastrointestinal systems.

35. B – Integrins
Margination of leukocytes involves the formation of weak and transient connections between leukocytes and the endothelium. These connections are mediated through selectin receptors expressed mainly by endothelial cells. Adhesion involves a strong bond between leukocytes and the endothelium and is formed between integrins expressed on leukocyte surfaces and adhesion molecules within the endothelium. Adhesion does not occur until activated by chemokines. Upregulation of selectins and endothelial adhesion molecules occurs during inflammation via mediators such as IL-1, TNF and histamine.

36. C – IgG
Chemokines is the name given to a family of chemotactic cytokines. IL-8 is an example of a chemokine released by macrophages to attract neutrophils. Leukotriene B4, platelet-activating factor and C5a all can also function chemotactically. IgG does not act directly as a chemotactic agent; however, certain bacteria (e.g. *Staphylococcus aureus*) can develop proteins to inhibit chemotaxis. The human body may then respond by producing antibodies to these proteins, again allowing chemotaxis to occur.

37. A – Ciliary ganglion
The preganglionic neurons originating from cranial nerve III synapse at the ciliary ganglion. These neurons arise from the Edinger–Westphal nucleus and terminate at the ciliary ganglion where postganglionic neurons continue to innervate the sphincter pupillae muscle of the iris and the ciliary muscle contained within the ciliary body.

38. B – Alveolar development continues until 2 years of age
A tracheal bud is formed from the foregut at 4–5 weeks' gestation. Formation of the major airways and bronchial tree continues to 16 weeks. After 16 weeks, the last generations of the lung periphery are formed, as well as epithelial differentiation and formation of the air–blood barrier. After 24 weeks, the lung starts to produce surfactants and this is of great clinical importance as it is only after this stage that the fetal lung is theoretically viable if the baby is born prematurely. Alveolar differentiation continues until 8–10 years of age.

39. D – The engulfment and digestion of solid particles by cells
Phagocytosis is the engulfment and digestion of solid particles by a cell. The intake of fluid into a cell by engulfment defines pinocytosis. Exocytosis is the process of excreting substances within a cell vesicle by

fusion with its cell membrane. Programmed cell death initiated from within the cell is apoptosis. Regrowth of blood vessels following injury can be described as angiogenesis or revascularization.

40. C – Type I alveolar cells are thick cells providing structural integrity to the surface lining
Type I alveolar cells are the surface for gas exchange and make up 90% of the alveolar surface lining. Though they play a role in structure, they are actually very thin to enable efficient gas exchange. Type II alveolar cells make up much less of the surface lining and produce surfactant, which is important in reducing surface tension.

41. D – Pterygopalatine ganglion
The preganglionic neurons originating from cranial nerve VII synapse at the pterygopalatine submandibular ganglion. These neurons originate in the superior salivary nucleus of the pons. From here, fibres leave the brainstem and pass to submandibular and pterygopalatine ganglia where they synapse with postganglionic fibres. Fibres from the pterygopalatine ganglion innervate the lacrimal gland and the nasal and oral mucous membranes, while those from the submandibular ganglion innervate salivary glands (submandibular and sublingual glands). The ciliary ganglion is the site for synapse for cranial nerve III, the coeliac ganglion forms part of the sympathetic division and the otic ganglion is the site for synapse for cranial nerve IX.

42. B – Cranial nerves VII/IX
Facial preganglionic parasympathetic neurons originate from the superior salivatory nucleus of the pons (second part of the brain stem) and exit the brain stem in the sensory root of the facial nerve, also known as nervus intermedius. From here they travel via their terminal ganglia (submandibular and pterygopalatine) *en route* to innervating the submandibular and sublingual salivary glands, lacrimal gland, and nasal and oral mucous membranes. Glossopharyngeal parasympathetic neurons originate from the inferior salivatory nucleus of the medulla (third part of the brain stem) and subsequently synapse with postganglionic neurons in the otic ganglion, which essentially innervates the parotid salivary gland.

43. A – Cough
Acute epiglottitis is the result of localized *Haemophilus influenzae* infection of the supraglottic larynx. It is a medical emergency as the inflamed epiglottis can cause complete airway obstruction. Symptoms and signs include fever, drooling and dysphagia. A cough is typically absent.

44. E – Increases secretions, peristalsis and relaxation of sphincter
Parasympathetic innervation of the gastrointestinal system results in increased secretions, stimulation of peristalsis and (generally) sphincter relaxation. Sympathetic innervation results in converse outcomes.

45. A – Leukotriene B4

Leukotriene B4 also aids neutrophil function through chemotaxis. It is antagonized by lipoxins. Thromboxane A2 causes vasoconstriction. Prostacyclin results in vasodilation. Prostaglandins are involved in increasing the sensation of pain and the production of fever.

46. B – Hot potato voice

A patient with a peritonsillar abscess (quinsy) may speak with a 'hot potato voice'. That is, they will speak as if there is a hot potato in their mouth! This is due to the distortion of vowels. Other symptoms may include pain, fever, malaise and headache.

47. D – Prostaglandin PGE2

Eicosanoids are molecules involved in cell signalling. They are produced as a result of the metabolism of arachidonic acid. Dependent upon their properties, eicosanoids can stimulate or inhibit features of inflammation. Prostaglandin E2 (PGE2) is known to increase the sensitivity of pain receptors and is involved in the development of fever. Leukotrienes B4 and C4, and thromboxane A2 cause vasoconstriction. Prostacyclin results in vasodilation.

48. A – Inhibition of cyclooxygenase 1 (COX-1)

The COX-1 enzyme is contained within the gastric mucosa and is involved in the production of prostaglandins that protect the stomach from gastric erosion. Ingestion of non-specific NSAIDs, such as aspirin or ibuprofen, inhibits both COX-1 and COX-2 enzymes. This therefore decreases the gastric protection provided by the mucosal prostaglandins, resulting in gastric ulcers. Glucocorticoids inhibit phospholipase A2 thereby inhibiting the release of arachidonic acid from cell membranes, with a resultant increased risk in gastric ulceration.

49. E – Nicotinic receptors

The regulation of gastric secretion and motility is via both neural and hormonal mechanisms. Gastric digestion occurs in three stages: cephalic, gastric and intestinal. In the cephalic stage, the cerebral cortex and feeding centre in the brain send impulses to the submucosal plexus via the parasympathetic preganglionic fibres in the vagus nerves. This ultimately results in impulses to the parietal cells, chief cells, mucous cells and gastric glands which release pepsinogen, hydrochloric acid, mucous and gastrin. These impulses also increase stomach motility. In the gastric stage, food distends the stomach and stimulates stretch receptors in its walls, and chemoreceptors monitor the pH of the stomach chyme. When these receptors are activated, they send impulses to the submucosal plexus which in turn activates parasympathetic and enteric fibres, leading to peristalsis (the intestinal stage). This is mediated by acetylcholine via nicotinic receptors.

50. E – Margination and rolling, adhesion of integrins to endothelium, diapedesis, chemotaxis towards site of injury

Margination describes the process by which leukocytes begin to flow closer to the endothelial surfaces within a vessel. Leukocytes are described as rolling when partial bonds between themselves and the endothelium slow their progress within a vessel. Adhesion involves the formation of strong bonds between leukocytes and the endothelium. Diapedesis is the outward passage of blood cells through an intact vessel wall. Chemotaxis involves the movement of blood cells along a chemical concentration gradient either towards or away from the source.

Questions Paper 8

1. Phagocytosis can induce the killing of engulfed bacteria in a number of ways. Which of the following substances would *not* be bactericidal?
   A. Elastase
   B. Hydrogen peroxide
   C. Hypochlorous free radical
   D. Nitric oxide free radical
   E. Reactive oxygen species

2. In which of the following are acid hydrolase enzymes found?
   A. Centrioles
   B. Cytoplasm
   C. Lysosomes
   D. Ribosomes
   E. Vacuoles

3. There is an overlap between the many functions of growth factors; however, which of the following statements best describes the prominent function(s) of platelet-derived growth factor?
   A. Angiogenesis
   B. Catalyses the actions of other growth factors
   C. Chemotaxis and proliferation of fibroblasts and smooth muscle cells
   D. Stimulates aggregation of platelets
   E. Stimulates epithelial proliferation

4. Which of the following is produced by the pyloric region of the stomach?
   A. Gastrin only
   B. Hydrochloric acid only
   C. Mucus, hydrochloric acid and pepsinogen
   D. Mucus only
   E. Pepsinogen only

5. Before migration of epithelial cells can occur to re-epithelialize an area following injury, which of the following needs to occur?
   A. Apoptosis of peripheral epithelial cells
   B. Cross-linked collagen deposition
   C. Detachment of desmosomes and hemidesmosomes
   D. Erythropoietin stimulation
   E. Formation of myosin filaments

6. A 77-year-old man has been newly diagnosed with atrial fibrillation. He has a past medical history of type 2 diabetes, hypertension and hyperthyroidism. What is the most appropriate anticoagulation regimen for him?
   A. Aspirin alone
   B. Aspirin and clopidogrel
   C. Aspirin, clopidogrel and warfarin
   D. Warfarin
   E. No anticoagulation required

7. Choose the option below which best describes the order in which cutaneous wounds undergo healing
   A. Formation of fibrin clot, inflammation and cell recruitment, proliferation and deposition of extracellular matrix, wound contraction
   B. Formation of fibrin clot, proliferation and deposition of extracellular matrix, inflammation and cell recruitment, wound contraction
   C. Inflammation and cell recruitment, formation of fibrin clot, proliferation and deposition of extracellular matrix, wound contraction
   D. Wound contraction, formation of fibrin clot, inflammation and cell recruitment, proliferation, deposition and organization of extracellular matrix
   E. Wound contraction, inflammation and cell recruitment, formation of fibrin clot, proliferation and deposition of extracellular matrix

8. In a healthy adult, the normal level for lactate in the blood is:
   A. 0 mmol/L
   B. <1 mmol/L
   C. <1.5 mmol/L
   D. <2 mmol/L
   E. <2.5 mmol/L

9. Acidaemia is best defined as which of the following?
   A. A decrease in the metabolic concentration of hydrogen ions
   B. A lactate level of 0.7 mmol/L
   C. A pH of 7.55
   D. An increase in the concentration of bicarbonate
   E. An increase in the metabolic concentration of hydrogen ions

10. Which of the following features is more prominent in healing by secondary intention, compared with healing by primary intention?
    A. Lack of infective contamination of the wound
    B. Minimal tissue destruction
    C. Quicker haemostasis
    D. Smaller scar
    E. Wound contraction

11. Vitamin C deficiency results in easily bleeding gums due to which one of the following?
    A. Decreased production of clotting factors
    B. Inhibition of collagen synthesis
    C. Inhibition of fibroblast proliferation
    D. Inhibition of vitamin K
    E. Thrombocytopaenia

12. Histologically, a granuloma can be described as an aggregate of:
    A. Cuboidal epithelium
    B. Eosinophils
    C. Epithelioid cells
    D. Mast cells
    E. Microglial cells

13. Which one of the following is *not* a common target for drug binding?
    A. Cell surface receptors
    B. Cytosol
    C. Enzymes
    D. Membrane ion channels
    E. Transport proteins

14. It may take over 10 days before a clinical response to antithyroid drugs is observed. Which of the options below is the main reason?
    A. Fast pharmacokinetic activity of antithyroid drugs
    B. Long action of inhibition of iodination of tyrosine
    C. Long half-life of T4
    D. Short half-life of T4
    E. Slow pharmacokinetic activity of antithyroid drugs

15. Which type of efferent motoneurons located in the spinal cord innervates the intrafusal muscle fibres within the muscle spindle?
    A. α (alpha) motoneurons
    B. β (beta) motoneurons
    C. δ (delta) motoneurons
    D. ε (epsilon) motoneurons
    E. γ (gamma) motoneurons

16. In a healthy adult the normal range for blood pH is:
    A. 6.95–7.25
    B. 7.15–7.35
    C. 7.15–7.55
    D. 7.36–7.44
    E. 7.55–7.65

17. In a healthy adult the normal range for the partial pressure of oxygen in an arterial blood gas taken in room air at sea level is:
    A. 5–8 kPa
    B. 8–10 kPa
    C. 10–12 kPa
    D. 12–13 kPa
    E. 13–14 kPa

18. Fibroblasts are essential for the formation of granulation tissue. Which of the following is *not* a constituent of granulation tissue?
    A. Collagen
    B. Elastin
    C. Fibronectin
    D. Glycosaminoglycans
    E. Interferon

19. Which type of collagen is most abundant in early granulation tissue?
    A. Type I
    B. Type II
    C. Type III
    D. Type IV
    E. Type V

20. In a healthy adult the normal range for the partial pressure of carbon dioxide in an arterial blood gas taken in room air at sea level is:
    A. 1.7–3 kPa
    B. 3.1–5 kPa
    C. 4.7–6 kPa
    D. 5.1–8 kPa
    E. 6.7–9 kPa

21. In a healthy adult, the normal range for hydrogen ions in the blood is:
    A. 20–28 nmol/L
    B. 24–32 nmol/L
    C. 36–44 nmol/L
    D. 40–48 nmol/L
    E. 44–52 nmol/L

22. A panic attack which leads to hyperventilation will characteristically lead to which acid–base imbalance?
    A. Metabolic acidosis with respiratory compensation
    B. Metabolic acidosis without respiratory compensation
    C. Metabolic alkalosis
    D. Respiratory acidosis
    E. Respiratory alkalosis

23. A blood film is requested for a patient with suspected chronic inflammation. The report included mention of 'rouleaux formation'. What serum blood test would indicate the same process?
    A. C-reactive protein
    B. Erythrocyte sedimentation rate
    C. Neutrophil count
    D. Platelet count
    E. White blood cell count

24. Non-steroidal anti-inflammatory drugs are used most extensively in the long-term management of which one of the following conditions?
    A. Paget disease
    B. Peptic ulcer disease
    C. Rheumatoid arthritis
    D. Systemic lupus erythematosus
    E. Ulcerative colitis

25. What is the traditional method of quantifying acid–base imbalance?
    A. Cockcroft–Gault formula
    B. Henderson–Hasselbalch equation
    C. Model for end-stage liver disease (MELD) score
    D. Rockall score
    E. Stewart physicochemical approach

26. A 34-year-old woman who is 26 weeks' pregnant is found to have a blood pressure of 160/80 mmHg at two consecutive antenatal appointments. She has no proteinuria. What is the most appropriate management option?
    A. Labetalol
    B. Losartan
    C. Methyldopa
    D. Ramipril
    E. Repeat the blood pressure at the next antenatal appointment and consider treatment if the blood pressure remains raised

27. Which of the following best describes the range of gastrointestinal side-effects which can potentially be induced by prolonged use of non-steroidal anti-inflammatory drugs?
    A. Diarrhoea, dyspepsia, gastritis, gastroduodenal ulceration, hepatitis
    B. Diarrhoea, dyspepsia, gastroduodenal ulceration, villous atrophy
    C. Dyspepsia, gastritis, gastroduodenal ulceration, intestinal stricture formation
    D. Gastroduodenal ulceration, gastritis, gastrointestinal polyp formation, nausea
    E. Hepatitis, duodenitis, anal fissure, gastroduodenal ulceration, dyspepsia

28. Which part of the duodenum is retroperitoneal?
    A. The distal section of the first part
    B. The second part
    C. The third part
    D. The fourth part
    E. All of the above

29. Which of the following is the most abundant cell type within the small intestine?
    A. Enterocytes
    B. Enteroendocrine cells
    C. Goblet cells
    D. Paneth cells
    E. Stem cells

30. A 32-year-old man requires long-term non-steroidal anti-inflammatory drugs (NSAIDs) for ankylosing spondylitis. Which of the following is the most suitable choice of drug to co-prescribe with his long-term NSAIDs?
    A. Loperamide
    B. Misoprostol
    C. Omeprazole
    D. Ranitidine
    E. Regular Gaviscon

31. Which of the following lists describes the main potential complications to both mother and baby of long-term non-steroidal anti-inflammatory drug administration in the later stages of pregnancy?
    A. Delayed onset and increased duration of labour, premature closure of ductus arteriosus, persistent pulmonary hypertension of the newborn
    B. Delayed onset of labour, meconium aspiration syndrome, respiratory distress syndrome
    C. Delayed onset of labour, premature closure of ductus arteriosus, meconium aspiration syndrome
    D. Premature onset of labour, delayed closure of ductus arteriosus, persistent pulmonary hypertension of the newborn
    E. Premature onset of labour, premature closure of ductus arteriosus, respiratory distress syndrome

32. Which of the following is the first-line management of a Caucasian hypertensive patient under the age of 55?
    A. Angiotensin-converting enzyme inhibitor
    B. Beta-blocker
    C. Calcium channel blocker
    D. Loop diuretic
    E. Thiazide diuretic

33. Which one of the following has an antiparallel orientation of its tetramers?
    A. Actin filaments
    B. Centrioles
    C. Intermediate filaments
    D. Microtubules
    E. None of the above

34. Which of the following cell types is classically found as the lining alveoli?
    A. Columnar epithelium
    B. Cuboidal epithelium
    C. Squamous epithelium
    D. Transitional epithelium
    E. None of the above

35. An obese 76-year-old man has a past medical history of type 2 diabe-
    tes mellitus diagnosed 29 years ago. On routine attendance to his GP
    for follow-up he is found to have a blood pressure of 166/92 mmHg.
    Which of the following management options is the most suitable?
    A. Amlodipine 5 mg
    B. Atenolol 50 mg
    C. Bendroflumethiazide 2.5 mg
    D. Ramipril 2.5 mg
    E. Ramipril 10 mg

36. A 64-year-old woman presents with a long history of hypertension.
    She has been on 10 mg amlodipine for many years, and on routine
    check-up her blood pressure is found to be 162/96 mmHg. A few weeks
    later it is re-checked and recorded as 164/92 mmHg. What is the most
    appropriate management option?
    A. Add bendroflumethiazide 2.5 mg
    B. Add bisoprolol 5 mg
    C. Add ramipril 5 mg
    D. Increase the amlodipine to 15 mg
    E. Stop amlodipine and change to ramipril 10 mg

37. Bone is derived from:
    A. Ectoderm
    B. Endoderm
    C. Mesoderm
    D. All of the above
    E. None of the above

38. Which of the following cell types classically has a basal nucleus?
    A. Columnar epithelium
    B. Cuboidal epithelium
    C. Squamous epithelium
    D. Transitional epithelium
    E. None of the above

39. Which of the following best describes a syndesmosis?
    A. A joint that allows the greatest mobility
    B. A joint with limited movement in which bones are covered by a hyaline cartilage on the articulating surface
    C. A joint with limited movement where the bones are joined by a hyaline cartilage
    D. A joint with limited movement where the bones are joined by an interosseous membrane
    E. A non-moveable joint where the bones are connected by bone tissue or dense connective tissue

40. Which of the following cell types contain granules which accumulate at the apical end of the cell?
    A. Enterocytes
    B. Enteroendocrine cells
    C. Goblet cells
    D. Paneth cells
    E. Stem cells

41. Keloid scars occur as a result of which of the following?
    A. Deposition of excessive amounts of collagen during scar formation
    B. Lack of vitamin C
    C. Reduced elastin deposition
    D. Reduced iron absorption
    E. Wounds penetrating deep into the dermis

42. Degradation of collagen and other extracellular components is commonly undertaken by which one of the following enzyme?
    A. Cyclooxygenase
    B. Elastase
    C. HMG-CoA reductase
    D. Matrix metalloproteinases
    E. Myeloperoxidase

43. Which part of the small intestine is characterized by the presence of plicae circulares?
    A. Caecum
    B. Duodenum
    C. Jejunum
    D. Proximal ileum
    E. Terminal ileum

44. Which one of the following organelles is studded with ribosomes?
    A. Golgi apparatus
    B. Mitochondria
    C. Nucleus
    D. Rough endoplasmic reticulum
    E. Smooth endoplasmic reticulum

45. Which one of the following maintains cell shape and enables cellular motion?
   A. Centrioles
   B. Cytoplasm
   C. Cytoskeleton
   D. Vacuoles
   E. Vesicles

46. Which of the following cell type is found in the bases of the intestinal crypts and contains large acidophilic granules?
   A. Enteroendocrine cells
   B. Enterocytes
   C. Goblet cells
   D. Paneth cells
   E. Stem cells

47. Which of the following drugs may be associated with a dry cough?
   A. Amiodarone
   B. Atenolol
   C. Isosorbide mononitrate
   D. Lisinopril
   E. Losartan

48. The normal range for actual bicarbonate in the blood is:
   A. 10–18 mmol/L
   B. 16–23 mmol/L
   C. 21–28 mmol/L
   D. 25–30 mmol/L
   E. 28–32 mmol/L

49. Which of the following is classically found as the apical layer of epithelium?
   A. Columnar epithelium
   B. Cuboidal epithelium
   C. Keratinized epithelium
   D. Squamous epithelium
   E. Transitional epithelium

50. What is the pH within the lumen of the stomach?
   A. 1–2
   B. 2–4
   C. 4–6
   D. 6–8
   E. 8–10

Answers Paper 8

1. A – Elastase
Reactive oxygen species (including hydrogen peroxide) and free radicals cause cellular damage to bacterial cells and their DNA, leading to death by apoptosis. Elastase is an enzyme that will degrade a microorganism once it has already been killed.

2. C – Lysosomes
Lysosomes are specialized vesicles containing acid hydrolase enzymes, which digest waste materials and cellular debris. Vesicles in general are bubbles of liquid within a cell that are used to store, transport or digest cellular products. A ribosome is responsible for the production of proteins from amino acids. They are divided into two subunits. The smaller of the two binds to messenger RNA (mRNA) and the larger to transfer RNA (tRNA). Vacuoles are enclosed compartments containing inorganic and organic molecules such as enzymes in solution. The cytoplasm is the part of the cell enclosed by the cell membrane. Centrioles are cylindrical structures made predominantly of the protein tubulin which are important in the organization of the cytoplasm and cell division.

3. C – Chemotaxis and proliferation of fibroblasts and smooth muscle cells
Platelet-derived growth factor (PDGF) is chemotactic to monocytes, fibroblasts and smooth muscle cells, and can be secreted by macrophages. Within healing tissues, it provides an important role in extracellular matrix formation via fibroblast and smooth muscle cell proliferation. Epithelial growth factor (EGF) stimulates epithelial proliferation. Angiogenesis is stimulated by vascular endothelial growth factor (VEGF) and fibroblast growth factor (FGF). PDGF shares some role in angiogenesis. Hypoxia is a strong stimulant of VEGF secretion. Insulin-like growth factor-1 (IGF-1) has synergistic actions with a number of factors. Adenosine diphosphate (ADP) and thromboxane A2, rather than PDGF, are involved in stimulating platelet aggregation.

4. D – Mucus only
In the cardia and pyloric regions of the stomach only mucus is produced. In the body and fundus of the stomach mucus, hydrochloric acid and pepsinogen are produced. Gastrin is only produced in the antrum.

5. C – Detachment of desmosomes and hemidesmosomes
Desmosomes are structures joining two adjacent epithelial cells. Hemidesmosomes anchor epithelial cells to the basement membrane.

Loosening of these connections is necessary in order for epithelial proliferation and migration over a wound. Migration occurs via actin microfilaments formed within the epithelial cells. Erythropoietin is a hormone released from the kidneys that stimulates the proliferation and maturation of red blood cells (erythrocytes). Organization of collagen and strengthening via crosslinks only occur later on in the healing process. Re-epithelialization is one of the first steps and aids granulation tissue formation.

6. D – Warfarin

Current guidelines suggest that patients with non-rheumatic atrial fibrillation are risk stratified prior to commencing anticoagulation treatment. To risk stratify patients, the CHA_2DS_2–VASc scoring system can be applied. The criteria are:

- C   Congestive heart failure
- H   Hypertension (BP > 140/90 or treated hypertension)
- A_2 Age ≥ 75
- D   Diabetes mellitus
- S_2 Prior stroke, TIA or thromboembolism
- V   Vascular disease (peripheral arterial disease, myocardial infarction)
- A   Age 65–74
- Sc   Sex category (i.e. female sex)

For each of the above criteria, one point is added, with the exception of age ≥75 and prior TIA/stroke/thromboembolism, where two points are added. In patients scoring 2 or above, oral anticoagulation should be started. Those who are at low risk (defined as a score of 0 in males or 1 in females) require no anticoagulation. Males scoring 1 are stratified as being at moderate risk, and oral anticoagulation is recommended. The patient in this scenario scores 4 points (2 for age, 1 for hypertension, 1 for diabetes), therefore he should be on warfarin.

7. A – Formation of fibrin clot, inflammation and cell recruitment, proliferation and deposition of extracellular matrix, wound contraction

Initially following injury to the skin, bleeding occurs, which stimulates vasoconstriction with activation of platelets and the clotting cascade. Vasodilation follows with inflammatory infiltrate, chemotaxis of inflammatory cells and removal of injured tissues. Proliferation then occurs and includes re-epithelialization, angiogenesis and collagen deposition. Wound contraction occurs at 1–2 weeks post-injury, followed by remodelling of collagen in order to regain the strength of the tissue.

8. D – <2 mmol/L

Lactate is constantly produced from pyruvate and constantly removed through gluconeogenesis and oxidation. It can be produced in higher amounts in critically ill patients, leading to acidaemia. Note that there is an increased mortality in critically ill patients with a raised lactate.

9. E – An increase in the metabolic concentration of hydrogen ions
Acidaemia is defined as a pH < 7.36, which correlates to a hydrogen concentration of greater than 44 nmol/L. Increased bicarbonate concentrations may increase the pH so it may become alkalotic. A pH of 7.55 is defined as alkalotic.

10. E – Wound contraction
Wounds that heal by secondary intention are those which result from more extensive tissue loss or require a longer healing period due to contamination with infective organisms. Wound contraction is undertaken by myofibroblasts and is needed for these larger wounds, and will usually result in a larger scar. Time to haemostasis may be prolonged with wounds healing by secondary intention, because there may have been greater destruction of vasculature.

11. B – Inhibition of collagen synthesis
The strength of collagen comes from its ability to form crosslinks. This process is dependent upon ascorbic acid (vitamin C).

12. C – Epithelioid cells
Epithelioid cells are activated macrophages which have changed in shape to resemble epithelial cells. They are an essential characteristic of granulomas.

13. B – Cytosol
A drug is a chemical that has the ability to alter the function/response of a molecule. A drug target is a physical and chemical structure that has the ability to interact with these chemicals. Any structure with this ability can be considered a drug target, and useful drug targets are those that can interact with chemicals and produce a clinically beneficial response. Common drug targets are as listed in the other options. Cytosol, the fluid substance of cytoplasm, is not a drug target though it may hold drug targets, such as nuclear receptors, in suspension.

14. C – Long half-life of T4
Thioureylenes, such as carbimazole and propylthiouracil, have a fast pharmacokinetic action, inhibiting tyrosine residue iodination on thyroglobulin and thus reducing thyroid hormone synthesis. The clinical response is still slow and may take several days however, due to the long half-life of T4 (thyroxine). Existing T4 will persist for some time and hence still cause clinical symptoms of hyperthyroidism. It is only when the existing hormones are eradicated that the fast pharmacokinetic action of antithyroid medications will produce a clinical effect.

15. E – γ (gamma) motoneurons
Somatic motoneurons are divided into only two types: alpha and gamma. The gamma-motoneurons innervate the intrafusal muscle fibres within the muscle spindle. They are used to regulate the sensitivity of the spindle

to muscle stretching. The alpha-motoneurons innervate extrafusal muscle fibres within the muscle. The alpha-motoneurons are often called the ventral horn neurons, as their cell body is located within the ventral horn of the spinal cord. They contribute to the muscle tone generated when a muscle is in a non-contracted state.

16. D – 7.36–7.44
The normal value for blood pH is between 7.36 and 7.44. Any lower or higher would indicate an acidaemia or alkalaemia, respectively.

17. D – 12–13 kPa
The normal arterial partial pressure of oxygen in room air at sea level is 12–13 kPa. This is the value for a young healthy adult, and the normal range will decrease with age.

18. E – Interferon
All of the components listed can be synthesized by fibroblasts; however, interferons do not contribute to the granulation tissue scaffolding formed within healing wounds. Interferons aid the immune system's response against viral infection.

19. C – Type III
Type I is the most abundant type of collagen within the skin, but type III collagen is most abundant in early granulation tissue. During maturation of collagen following cutaneous injury, type III collagen is replaced with type I.

20. C – 4.7–6 kPa
In a normal young healthy adult, the normal range for partial pressure of carbon dioxide in an arterial blood gas taken at sea level when breathing room air is 4.7–6 kPa. If there is a constant metabolic rate, the $PaCO_2$ is determined only by ventilation. If hypoventilating, the $PaCO_2$ will rise, leading to a respiratory acidosis, and if hyperventilating the $PaCO_2$ will decrease, leading to a respiratory alkalosis.

21. C – 36–44 nmol/L
The normal range of hydrogen ions in the blood is between 36 and 44 nmol/L. This equates to the normal pH range of between 7.36 and 7.44.

22. E – Respiratory alkalosis
Hyperventilation will lead to the loss of carbon dioxide, which leads to the loss of water. These have dissociated from H_2CO_3. $HCO_3^- + H^+ \rightleftharpoons H_2CO_3$ and $H_2CO_3 \rightleftharpoons CO_2 + H_2O$. The loss of hydrogen ions, as seen in these equations, results in an alkalosis.

23. B – Erythrocyte sedimentation rate
When fibrinogen binds to erythrocytes, it causes them to form aggregates, or *rouleaux*. This increases the rate at which they sediment when compared to individual red blood cells, hence increasing the erythrocyte sedimentation rate. An abundance of fibrinogen occurs with inflammatory states.

24. C – Rheumatoid arthritis
NSAIDs are used in a wide range of chronic inflammatory disorders, and therefore their use in rheumatology is prominent. Their largest single use is probably in the management of rheumatoid arthritis, a condition in which excess tumour necrosis factor (TNF)-α production leads to joint destruction, although they are used in conditions such as systemic lupus erythematosus to a lesser extent. NSAIDs should be co-prescribed with a proton-pump inhibitor if used long term to protect the gastroduodenal mucosa from ulceration. Regular monitoring of renal function should also be performed. The availability of disease-modifying therapies and biologic agents such as infliximab (anti-TNF-α monoclonal antibodies) has significantly reduced the need for long-term NSAID use.

25. B – Henderson–Hasselbalch equation
The Henderson–Hasselbalch equation is used to find the equilibrium pH in acid–base reactions. The Stewart approach is a newer method of acid–base analysis, with the focus on electron neutrality versus pH control. The Cockcroft–Gault formula is for creatinine clearance, MELD score is for assessment of end-stage liver disease and the Rockall score is used to identify patients at risk of an adverse outcome following acute upper gastrointestinal bleeding.

26. A – Labetalol
This patient has gestational hypertension, which is defined as new hypertension presenting after 20 weeks' gestation without significant proteinuria. First-line treatment is oral labetalol with the aim of keeping the diastolic blood pressure between 80 and 90 mmHg and the systolic blood pressure under 150 mmHg. With a blood pressure as high as 160/80 mmHg, the patient in this scenario would also require admission to hospital. Ramipril is contraindicated during pregnancy and breastfeeding, as is losartan. Methyldopa is no longer the agent of choice but can be used if there is a contraindication to beta blockers, such as asthma. The significance of the absence of proteinuria is extremely important in a pregnant woman to ensure that this is not pre-eclampsia.

27. A – Diarrhoea, dyspepsia, gastritis, gastroduodenal ulceration, hepatitis
Although the range of gastrointestinal side-effects caused by NSAIDs is diverse, NSAIDs are not known to be associated with polyp formation, villous atrophy, anal fissures or stricture formation.

28. E – All of the above
Apart from the first 2 cm of the first part of the duodenum, it is all retroperitoneal and consequently immobile.

29. A – Enterocytes
Enterocytes are the most abundant cell type in the small intestine. They are tall columnar cells with microvilli and a basal nucleus. They are specialized cells and serve to absorb and transport substances in and out

of the lumen. They have a short lifespan, which allows for the continual wear and tear of the intestinal mucosa.

30. C – Omeprazole

With long-term NSAID therapy, gastroprotection against ulceration is crucial. The most suitable choice in the vast majority of patients is a proton-pump inhibitor, such as omeprazole. H_2-receptor blockers, such as ranitidine, protect against duodenal ulcers but have little protective effect against gastric ulcers. Misoprostol is an alternative, although diarrhoea and abdominal pain are frequent and troublesome side-effects.

31. A – Delayed onset and increased duration of labour, premature closure of ductus arteriosus, persistent pulmonary hypertension of the newborn

The main potential complications of long-term NSAID use in later pregnancy are a delayed onset and increased duration of labour, premature closures of the ductus arteriosus and persistent pulmonary hypertension of the newborn. NSAIDs inhibit prostaglandin synthesis, which is the mechanism by which long-term use in the third trimester results in these complications. Prostaglandins are important in promoting myometrial contractions and therefore in the initiation of labour. A fall in prostaglandin levels at birth is in part responsible for contraction of the vascular smooth muscle of the ductus arteriosus wall and therefore its closure. NSAIDs reverse both of these processes, hence delayed onset and prolonged duration of labour and premature closure of the ductus arteriosus.

32. A – Angiotensin-converting enzyme inhibitor

Current guidelines suggest that patients under the age of 55, who are non-black, should be treated with an ACE inhibitor. Beta-blockers have fallen out of favour for managing hypertension as they were found not to reduce the incidence of mortality. Use of either a calcium channel blocker or diuretic is recommended for patients who are over the age of 55, or who are black.

33. C – Intermediate filaments

Intermediate filaments have an antiparallel orientation of their tetramers and consequently, unlike other filaments, are not polarized. Actin filaments are assembled into two arrangements. Bundles can be composed of polar (all barbed ends point to the same end of the bundle) or non-polar (barbed ends point towards both ends) arrays of filaments. Microtubules are polymers of α- and β-tubulin dimers. The tubulin dimers polymerize end-to-end in protofilaments.

34. C – Squamous epithelium

Squamous cells are thin flat cells which fit closely together. Their nuclei are flattened and elliptical. Squamous cells classically line the alveoli to allow passive diffusion. Cuboidal cells appear square in cross-section and are commonly found in secretive or absorptive tissue, such as in the secretory pancreas. Columnar cells are elongated with basal nuclei. They form the lining of the stomach and intestines. Transitional epithelium (urothelium) is a type of tissue which has the ability to contract and expand. They can appear to look like cuboidal or columnar cells. This ability to change shape allows the cells to accommodate fluctuations in volume within the bladder.

35. D – Ramipril 2.5 mg

Guidelines suggest that diabetic patients should have a target blood pressure of <130/80 mmHg. While there will be a beneficial effect of reducing the blood pressure by any means, ACE inhibitors confer additional benefit by reducing microalbuminuria in diabetic patients. A starting dose of ramipril 10 mg would be excessive. Renal function must be monitored and the dose gradually titrated up to the maximum tolerated dose for maximal cardiovascular benefit.

36. A – Add bendroflumethiazide 2.5 mg

The maximum licensed dose of amlodipine is 10 mg. Both ramipril and bisoprolol are not the appropriate next management steps in accordance with current NICE guidelines. It is never recommended to stop a medication simply because optimum blood pressure has not been achieved, merely to swap it for a different one. NICE guidelines recommend the addition of a diuretic to an existing calcium channel blocker in hypertensive individuals over the age of 55, or who are black.

37. C – Mesoderm

Bone and cartilage are some of the many tissues derived from the mesoderm. The mesoderm is one of the primary germ layers and also gives rise to muscle, connective tissue and the mid-layer of the skin.

38. A – Columnar epithelium

Columnar cells are elongated with basal nuclei. They form the lining of the stomach and intestines. Squamous cells are thin flat cells which fit closely together. Their nuclei are flattened and elliptical. Squamous cells classically line the alveoli to allow passive diffusion. Cuboidal cells appear square in cross-section and are commonly found in secretive or absorptive tissue, such as in the secretory pancreas. Transitional epithelium (urothelium) is a type of tissue which has the ability to contract and expand. These cells may look like cuboidal or columnar cells. This ability to change shape allows the cells to accommodate fluctuations in volume within the bladder.

39. D – A joint with limited movement where the bones are joined by an interosseous membrane

An interosseous membrane, such as the tibiofibular membrane, is an example of a syndesmosis joint (i.e. a joint with limited movement joined by connective tissue). A synchondrosis joint has limited movement and is connected by hyaline cartilage, such as the joints between the ribs and the sternum. A symphysis is a joint where there is limited movement but the bones involved have hyaline cartilage on their articulating surface, such as the pubic symphysis. Finally, a diarthrosis joint allows greater mobility and also has a synovial fluid contained within the joint, for example the knee.

40. C – Goblet cells

Goblet cells are the second most common epithelial cell type in the gastrointestinal tract. They increase in number along the length of the intestine. They contain mucous granules which accumulate at the apical (luminal) end of the cell, thus giving the cell a goblet-shaped appearance. The mucus secreted facilitates the passage of material through the bowel.

41. A – Deposition of excessive amounts of collagen during scar formation

Keloid formation occurs as a result of excessive collagen deposition, and the scar that forms can extend beyond the original limits of the wound. Keloid formation is more common in people of black ethnicity. Even a relatively superficial epithelial injury can result in a keloid scar in a susceptible individual.

42. D – Matrix metalloproteinases

Matrix metalloproteinases (MMPs) are proteolytic enzymes that degrade collagen, elastin, fibronectin, laminin and glycosaminoglycans.

43. C – Jejunum

The plicae circulares, or valvulae conniventes, are large flaps which project into the lumen of the bowel. They are present throughout the small intestine but are most prominent in the jejunum. They extend transversely for up to two-thirds of the circumference of the lumen. Plicae circulares slow the passage of food and increase the surface area for absorption.

44. D – Rough endoplasmic reticulum

Rough endoplasmic reticulum is so called because of the presence of ribosomes bound to its surface. They are not a stable part of the structure as they are constantly being released from the membrane.

45. C – Cytoskeleton

The cytoskeleton is a dynamic structure which is able to maintain cellular shape and allow cellular motion. It is also important in the movement of vesicles and organelles. Vesicles are bubbles of liquid within a cell and are used to store, transport or digest cellular products. A ribosome is responsible for the production of proteins from amino acids. They are divided into two subunits. The smaller of the two binds to messenger RNA (mRNA) and the larger to transfer RNA (tRNA). Vacuoles are enclosed compartments containing inorganic and organic molecules such as enzymes in solution. Cytoplasm is the part of the cell enclosed by the cell membrane. Centrioles are cylindrical structures made predominantly of the protein tubulin which are important in the organization of the cytoplasm and cell division.

46. D – Paneth cells
Paneth cells are found throughout the intestinal tract. They contain zinc and lysozyme. They are thought to contribute to host defence and the regulation of intestinal flora. Enterocytes are the main cells of the intestine, goblet cells secrete mucous and stem cells are able to become any type of intestinal cell.

47. D – Lisinopril
Angiotensin-converting enzyme (ACE) inhibitors are associated with a dry cough in some individuals. This is thought to be due to bradykinin in the lungs, as ACE normally metabolizes bradykinin. It is advised to transfer patients suffering with this side-effect to an angiotensin receptor blocker, such as losartan.

48. C – 21–28 mmol/L
The normal range for circulating actual bicarbonate is approximately 21–28 mmol/L. This is the value for a young healthy adult kept under standard conditions, i.e. at 37°C and with a $PaCO_2$ of 5.3 kPa. This provides normalized respiratory conditions which eliminate changes in bicarbonate resulting from potentially abnormal patient respiration. Also note that the normal range for standard bicarbonate is 21–27 mmol/L.

49. C – Keratinized epithelium
Keratinized epithelium is usually the most apical layer of epithelium. These cells are dead and lose their nucleus and cytoplasm. They contain keratin which is a tough, fibrous and waterproof protein.

50. A – 1–2
Within the stomach approximately 2 L of acid is produced per day. This equates to approximately 150 nmol/L hydrogen ions. Therefore the pH in the lumen of the stomach is low – between 1 and 2 – compared with between 6 and 7 at the epithelial surface.

Questions Paper 9

1. Which of the following is secreted by gastric chief cells?
   A. Gastrin
   B. Intrinsic factor
   C. Pepsinogen
   D. Secretin
   E. None of the above

2. Which of the following is *not* a cause of post-renal kidney injury?
   A. Benign prostatic hyperplasia
   B. Dehydration
   C. Invasive pelvic tumour
   D. Renal calculi
   E. Urethral stricture

3. Which one of the following statements regarding the body fluid compartments is *incorrect*?
   A. Extracellular fluid is further divided into interstitial fluid and plasma.
   B. Extracellular sodium is higher than intracellular sodium.
   C. Interstitial fluid has a higher protein content than plasma.
   D. The concentration of potassium is higher in intracellular than extracellular fluid.
   E. The intracellular compartment has approximately double the volume of the extracellular compartment.

4. From which part(s) of the stomach is intrinsic factor secreted?
   A. Antrum
   B. Body
   C. Cardia
   D. Fundus
   E. Fundus and body

5. Which of the following is the first phase of gastric secretion?
   A. Cephalic phase
   B. Gastric phase
   C. Intestinal phase
   D. Secretory phase
   E. None of the above

6. The sinoatrial node usually derives its blood supply from which of the following coronary arteries?
    A. Diagonal artery
    B. Left anterior descending artery
    C. Left circumflex artery
    D. Obtuse marginal artery
    E. Right coronary artery

7. By which of the following mechanisms do loop diuretics promote diuresis?
    A. Antidiuretic hormone inhibition
    B. Carbonic anhydrase inhibition
    C. H^+/K^+ transporter inhibition
    D. Na^+/H^+ pump stimulation
    E. $Na^+/K^+/2Cl^-$ co-transport inhibition

8. Which one of the following statements regarding urine formation by the kidney is correct?
    A. Primary filtration occurs at the proximal tubule.
    B. Reabsorption takes place at Bowman's capsule.
    C. Secretion of electrolytes occurs into the glomerulus.
    D. Sodium is reabsorbed by passive diffusion, along with potassium and chloride ions.
    E. The volume of water reabsorbed from the collecting duct depends on the presence of antidiuretic hormone.

9. A 7-year-old boy is taken to his GP by his concerned mother regarding a sore throat. The GP diagnoses a minor viral upper respiratory tract infection. However, an incidental finding of a 'machine-like murmur' just below the left clavicle is heard. What is the diagnosis?
    A. Aortic coarctation
    B. Atrial septal defect
    C. Normal physiological murmur
    D. Patent ductus arteriosus
    E. Ventricular septal defect

10. Renin is secreted by the kidney in response to reduced renal perfusion. Which one of the following statements best describes the action of this hormone?
    A. It causes vasodilatation of the glomerulus.
    B. It cleaves angiotensinogen to aldosterone.
    C. It converts angiotensinogen to angiotensin I.
    D. It converts angiotensin I to angiotensin II.
    E. It reduces blood pressure by promoting diuresis.

11. A 64-year-old man who recently retired from work in the dye industry presents with painless haematuria. Biopsy at cystoscopy diagnoses bladder carcinoma. Which of the following is the most common type of urothelial cancer?
    A. Adenocarcinoma
    B. Columnar cell carcinoma
    C. Myosarcoma
    D. Squamous cell carcinoma
    E. Transitional cell carcinoma

12. Parietal cells produce which of the following?
    A. Gastric acid
    B. Gastrin
    C. Pepsin
    D. Pepsinogen
    E. Secretin

13. Which of the following cells secrete intrinsic factor?
    A. Chief cells
    B. Enteroendocrine cells
    C. Mucous cells
    D. Parietal cells
    E. None of the above

14. Which of the following is *not* a cause of increased plasma urea?
    A. Acute renal failure
    B. Dehydration
    C. High-protein diet
    D. Pregnancy
    E. Upper gastrointestinal bleeding

15. Which one of the following is *not* a function of the kidney?
    A. Elimination of drugs and metabolic waste products
    B. Regulation of acid–base balance
    C. Regulation of blood pressure
    D. Regulation of erythrocyte production
    E. Stimulation of the innate immune response

16. Which one of the following statements regarding the process of apoptosis is correct?
    A. Apoptosis hinders wound healing.
    B. Apoptosis is only initiated via a mitochondrial-dependent intrinsic pathway.
    C. Apoptosis is only initiated via extrinsic mechanisms that are triggered by death receptors on the cell surface.
    D. Apoptosis requires ATP as an energy source.
    E. Apoptosis results in the influx of ions and water causing cell lysis.

17. The volume of anatomical dead space in an average adult is:
    A. 50 mL
    B. 150 mL
    C. 300 mL
    D. 500 mL
    E. 1 L

18. Which one of the following statements regarding the role of the kidneys in acid–base balance is correct?
    A. A plasma pH of 7.25 will be compensated by reduced renal HCO_3^- reabsorption.
    B. Hydrogen ion secretion occurs via H^+-ATPase and Na^+/H^+ co-transporters.
    C. Renal compensation occurs acutely (within hours) in respiratory alkalosis.
    D. Respiratory acidosis results in a reduction of H^+ secretion by the renal tubules and reduced reabsorption of HCO_3^-.
    E. The Henderson–Hasselbalch equation is used to calculate renal perfusion in disorders of acid–base balance.

19. Which one of the following factors decreases the volume of anatomical dead space?
    A. Bronchodilators
    B. Head of subject tilted forward
    C. Increasing size of subject
    D. Increasing tidal volume of subject
    E. Younger age of subject

20. Which one of the following statements regarding the role of apoptosis is correct?
    A. Self-reacting B-cells undergo apoptosis in the thymus more commonly than T-cells.
    B. T-cells that react with self major histocompatibility complex proteins are destroyed by apoptosis in the thymus in a process called 'peripheral tolerance'.
    C. T-cells with antigen receptors to 'self-antigens' are destroyed by apoptosis in the thymus.
    D. T-cells with antigen receptors undergo necrosis in a process called 'negative selection'.
    E. Tolerance ensures that external 'foreign' stimuli do not elicit an immune response after foetal life.

21. Optimal gas exchange by the respiratory tract is met by the following characteristics, *except*:
    A. The tract has a large gas permeable surface area.
    B. The tract has an effective system for gas delivery to the alveoli.
    C. The tract is able to warm and humidify inhaled gases.

D. The tract is open to the atmosphere.
E. There is a small deoxygenated blood supply in close relation to the gas permeable surface.

22. What is the tidal volume in an average adult?
    A. 250 mL
    B. 500 mL
    C. 1000 mL
    D. 1500 mL
    E. 2000 mL

23. Which vessel supplies approximately 75% of the liver's blood?
    A. Cystic artery
    B. Hepatic artery
    C. Hepatic vein
    D. Portal vein
    E. Splenic artery

24. Which of the following values are *incorrect*?
    A. Functional residual capacity is around 2.7 L in the average adult.
    B. Intrapleural pressure ranges from −0.5 to −1.0 cmH$_2$O.
    C. Residual volume is around 1.2 L in the average adult.
    D. Tidal volume is around 0.5 L in the average adult.
    E. Total lung capacity is around 4.8 L in the average adult.

25. The normal P–R interval on an ECG should be:
    A. <0.12 seconds
    B. 0.12–0.2 seconds
    C. 0.38–0.42 seconds
    D. >0.2 seconds
    E. >0.4 seconds

26. Which vessel is usually found in Calot's triangle?
    A. Cystic artery
    B. Hepatic artery
    C. Hepatic vein
    D. Portal vein
    E. Splenic artery

27. The T wave of an ECG represents:
    A. Atrial depolarization
    B. Atrial repolarization
    C. Ventricular depolarization
    D. Ventricular filling
    E. Ventricular repolarization

28. Which of the following is an example of a zymogen?
    A. Gastrin
    B. Intrinsic factor

C. Pepsinogen
D. Secretin
E. None of the above

29. The main spread of depolarization, from the inside out through the base of the ventricles, describes which of the following?
    A. P wave
    B. Q wave
    C. R wave
    D. S wave
    E. T wave

30. A slim 66-year-old woman who is a lifelong smoker presents to the emergency department with a cough productive of yellow sputum and left-sided chest pain. She looks short of breath and has oxygen saturation levels of 84% on air. Her JVP is not elevated and she has no peripheral oedema. The rest of her observations are as follows: temperature 38.1°C, BP 100/56 mmHg, pulse 110/min and irregular. A routine ECG is done. What would you expect the ECG to show?
    A. A completely normal trace
    B. Atrial fibrillation with globally small complexes
    C. Changes consistent with an acute myocardial infarction
    D. Electrical alternans
    E. $S_I Q_{III} T_{III}$

31. A 15-year-old girl is found to have a difference between her arm and leg blood pressures, with the arm pressures being markedly higher. She is also noted to have a wide carrying angle, webbed neck and widely spaced nipples. What is the most likely cause of the blood pressure difference?
    A. Aortic coarctation
    B. Aortic stenosis
    C. Dissection of the thoracic aorta
    D. Mitral regurgitation
    E. Congestive heart failure

32. Enterochromaffin-like cells release which of the following?
    A. Acetylcholine
    B. Gastric acid
    C. Histamine
    D. Serotonin
    E. None of the above

33. A 44-year-old woman is known to have aortic coarctation and refused corrective surgery many years ago. What abnormality might be found on a chest X-ray?
    A. A grossly enlarged heart
    B. An enlarged aortic knuckle

C. Large bilateral pleural effusions
D. Rib notching
E. No abnormality

34. Which of the following is an α_1-receptor blocker that directly antagonizes sympathetic control of vascular tone?
   A. Diazoxide
   B. Doxazosin
   C. Methyldopa
   D. Minoxidil
   E. Ramipril

35. The loss of elasticity with age in which vessel type can lead to an increase in systolic blood pressure?
   A. Arteriole
   B. Artery
   C. Capillary
   D. Vein
   E. Venule

36. Which of the following drugs is a glycoprotein IIb/IIIa receptor antagonist?
   A. Aspirin
   B. Clopidogrel
   C. Dipyridamole
   D. Epoprostenol
   E. Tirofiban

37. Which pulse is found behind the knee?
   A. Brachial
   B. Carotid
   C. Femoral
   D. Popliteal
   E. Radial

38. Which of the following gives good analgesia as the first-line treatment of colicky abdominal pain?
   A. Diamorphine
   B. Fentanyl
   C. Hyoscine
   D. Morphine
   E. Tramadol

39. Which of the following is *not* a branch of the internal pudendal artery?
   A. Deep artery of the clitoris/penis
   B. Dorsal artery of the clitoris/penis
   C. Inferior rectal artery
   D. Perineal arteries
   E. Superior gluteal artery

40. What is the total volume of cerebrospinal fluid?
    A. 15 mL
    B. 50 mL
    C. 150 mL
    D. 500 mL
    E. 1000 mL

41. Which one of the following options is true regarding the anatomy of the fourth ventricle?
    A. Connected to the lateral ventricles via the foramina of Luschka
    B. Connected to the third ventricle via the foramen of Magendie
    C. Located in the midbrain
    D. Located in the pons anterior to the cerebellum
    E. Medial to the thalamus

42. During the first trimester of pregnancy, what happens to the cardiac output?
    A. Decreases by 10%–15%
    B. Decreases by 30%–40%
    C. Increases by 10%–15%
    D. Increases by 30%–40%
    E. Remains unchanged

43. Which of the following is the most common isolated congenital heart defect?
    A. Atrial septal defect
    B. Coarctation of the aorta
    C. Patent ductus arteriosus
    D. Tricuspid atresia
    E. Ventricular septal defect

44. Where is cerebrospinal fluid produced?
    A. Arachnoid villi
    B. Choroid plexus
    C. Foramina of Luschka
    D. Spinal cord
    E. Subarachnoid space

45. Which one of the following factors make direct current cardioversion less likely to be successful?
    A. Alcohol-induced atrial fibrillation in a young patient
    B. Atrial flutter
    C. Enlarged left atrium
    D. Short duration since onset
    E. Underlying infection

46. What does the Q-wave on an ECG represent?
    A. Atrial depolarization
    B. Atrial repolarization
    C. Depolarization at the bundle of His
    D. Repolarization at the bundle of His
    E. Ventricular repolarization

47. Which of the following is the site of absorption of cerebrospinal fluid?
    A. Arachnoid villi
    B. Choroid plexus
    C. Foramina of Luschka
    D. Spinal cord
    E. Subarachnoid space

48. Which of the following cranial nerves (CN) is responsible for facial sensation?
    A. CN II
    B. CN III
    C. CN IV
    D. CN V
    E. CN IX

49. Which of the following is the branch of the superior mesenteric artery that gives rise to the appendiceal artery?
    A. Ileocolic artery
    B. Left colic artery
    C. Marginal artery of Drummond
    D. Middle colic artery
    E. Right colic artery

50. Which one of the following statements regarding the process of necrosis is correct?
    A. Failure of necrosis can lead to malignant tumour growth.
    B. Necrosis is a component of normal cell growth and development.
    C. Necrosis is a tightly regulated, active process which prevents cell proliferation and malignant tumour growth.
    D. Necrosis is accidental cell death which results in the swelling of cells and organelles, and ultimately cell lysis.
    E. Necrosis was first discovered as a normal component of developing embryos.

Answers Paper 9

1. C – Pepsinogen
Gastric chief cells secrete pepsinogen, gastric lipase and rennin. Gastrin and secretin stimulate the secretion of pepsinogen. They work in relation to parietal cells in the conversion of pepsinogen to pepsin. Chief cells contain a high concentration of rough endoplasmic reticulum.

2. B – Dehydration
Acute renal failure can be divided into three types: pre-renal, intrinsic and post-renal. Pre-renal failure is caused by impaired perfusion of the kidneys. This may be secondary to heart failure (causing reduced cardiac output and hypotension) or caused by hypovolaemia, secondary to dehydration or severe haemorrhage. Intrinsic renal failure occurs when there is a damage to the kidney itself, e.g. glomerulonephritis. Nephrotoxic drugs (e.g. gentamicin) can cause tubular necrosis, which results in intrinsic renal failure. Finally, post-renal failure results from obstruction of the urinary system distal to the renal calyces (e.g. renal calculi, benign prostatic hyperplasia, strictures or tumours).

3. C – Interstitial fluid has a higher protein content than plasma
Body water makes up approximately 60% of body weight and is divided into extracellular (20%) and intracellular compartments (40%). Extracellular fluid is split into interstitial fluid and plasma, which are separated only by the thin, permeable capillary membrane. The larger plasma proteins cannot pass through this membrane, thus plasma protein content is higher than that of the interstitial fluid. The electrolyte composition of the extracellular and intracellular compartments is usually well maintained. The osmotic gradient between the two compartments controls the distribution of fluid between the two. Sodium concentrations are higher in the extracellular fluid (approximately 139–145 mmol/L), while potassium is higher intracellularly (approximately 140 mmol/L, compared with 3.6–5 mmol/L extracellularly).

4. C – Cardia
A zymogen is an inactive enzyme precursor. Pepsinogen is an example of this and requires a biochemical change to alter the configuration and reveal the active site of the enzyme. Pepsinogen is activated by the hydrochloric acid released from parietal cells. The autocatalytic reaction which ensues produces pepsin, which acts upon the carbon bonds of aromatic amino acids.

167

5. A – Cephalic phase

The cephalic phase is the conditioned phase where food is thought about, smelt and tasted. This stimulates the vagus nerve and leads to the release of acetylcholine, resulting in histamine release. Histamine stimulates the release of gastrin and this leads to the production of gastric acid. When food arrives in the stomach, stretch receptors and chemoreceptors are stimulated. This is the second (gastric) phase. Somatostatin is released to lower the pH. The third is the intestinal phase, where fats in the duodenum lead to the release of cholecystokinin (CCK) and gastric inhibitory peptide. CCK stimulates chief cells to release pepsinogen and gastric inhibitory polypeptide (GIP) inhibits acid production.

6. E – Right coronary artery

The right coronary artery (RCA) supplies the sinoatrial node (SAN) in 60% of individuals. The other 40% derive the blood supply to the SAN from the left circumflex artery. Occlusion of the RCA results in inferior ischaemic changes on electrocardiography. This is because the RCA provides blood supply to the right ventricle which forms most of the inferior border of the heard. Arrhythmias may arise if the SAN is involved downstream of an RCA occlusion.

7. E – Na$^+$/K$^+$/2Cl$^-$ co-transport inhibition

Furosemide is a loop diuretic frequently used in the management of hypertension. It is also effective in treating peripheral and pulmonary oedema, secondary to heart failure. Loop diuretics act by inhibiting chloride reabsorption in the ascending limb of the loop of Henle. This leads to natriuresis and, because water follows sodium, diuresis. Inhibition of the Na$^+$/K$^+$/2Cl$^-$ co-transporter means that potassium ions are also excreted, which can lead to hypokalaemia if potassium supplements are not given.

8. E – The volume of water reabsorbed from the collecting duct depends on the presence of antidiuretic hormone

The formation of urine begins with glomerular filtration. The glomerulus is a network of capillaries encapsulated by Bowman's capsule. After the glomerular filtrate enters Bowman's capsule, it passes into the proximal tubule. The proximal tubule is made up of cuboidal epithelium with an apical membrane of microvilli that increases the surface area for reabsorption. The active transport of sodium underlies the reabsorption of other solutes, including amino acids, glucose and electrolytes. Electrolytes such as potassium and hydrogen ions are actively secreted into the tubule. Distal to the proximal tubule, the filtrate enters the descending limb of the loop of Henle. This portion of the renal tubule is highly permeable to water, causing water to move out and into the hyperosmotic interstitium. The ascending limb is relatively impermeable to water and so it remains in the tubule, while sodium, chloride and potassium ions are reabsorbed. This results in hypotonic tubular fluid. Active transport of sodium and chloride into the interstitium creates a hyperosmolar medullary inter-stitium. The permeability of the late distal tubule and collecting duct is dependent on the secretion of antidiuretic hormone (ADH). This allows tight hypothalamic–pituitary control of extracellular fluid osmolarity.

9. D – Patent ductus arteriosus

This is a relatively typical presentation of a patent ductus arteriosus (PDA). The majority of children with a PDA are asymptomatic, and the 'machine-like murmur' is picked up as an incidental finding. In normal physiology, the ductus arteriosus closes in the first month after birth but is likely to remain patent for longer in premature babies. Prostaglandin release is thought to keep the duct patent, and pharmacological closure can some-times be achieved with administration of the NSAID indomethacin.

10. C – It converts angiotensinogen to angiotensin I

The renin–angiotensin–aldosterone (RAA) axis plays a vital role in the regulation of blood pressure and fluid balance. Angiotensinogen is con-verted to angiotensin I by renin, which is secreted by the juxtaglomerular apparatus of the kidney in response to reduced perfusion. Angiotensin II is formed from angiotensin I by angiotensin converting enzyme (ACE). Angiotensin II works to increase blood pressure by promoting vasocon-striction and aldosterone secretion from the adrenal cortex. Together, these two hormones increase reabsorption of sodium and water, thus increasing blood volume and raising blood pressure. Many antihyper-tensives act on this system and reduce blood pressure by inhibiting the RAA axis at various stages. For example, ramipril and enalapril inhibit ACE, while spironolactone inhibits aldosterone. Angiotensin II receptor blockers (e.g. losartan) can also be used to block the RAA pathway in the management of hypertension.

11. E – Transitional cell carcinoma

Painless haematuria is a common presentation of bladder malignancy. Predisposing factors include occupation in the dye industry (exposure to benzidine and α-naphthylamine), smoking and drugs, such as cyclophos-phamide. Over 90% of bladder cancers are of transitional cell origin.

12. A – Gastric acid

Parietal cells produce gastric (hydrochloric) acid in response to hista-mine, acetylcholine and gastrin. The cells themselves contain canaliculi from which gastric acid is secreted by active transport into the stomach. (Note that this concentration gradient is the steepest in the human body.) They also produce intrinsic factor which is required for the absorption of vitamin B_{12}.

13. D – Parietal cells

Parietal cells produce gastric acid in response to histamine, acetylcholine and gastrin. The cells themselves contain canaliculi from which gastric acid is secreted by active transport into the stomach. They also produce intrinsic factor which is required for the absorption of vitamin B_{12}.

14. D – Pregnancy
Plasma urea and creatinine rise in response to a reduction in the glomerular filtration rate (GFR), which may be caused by damage of the glomeruli or poor renal perfusion. Urea and creatinine do not rise above the normal range until GFR declines by approximately 50–60%. Increased production of urea occurs with a high-protein diet, increased muscle mass and catabolic states (e.g. cancer, surgery or trauma). Upper gastrointestinal bleeding also causes an increase in urea because of absorption and breakdown of blood proteins released into the gut. GFR usually increases in pregnancy (by up to 50%), which tends to lower the concentration of plasma urea.

15. E – Stimulation of the innate immune response
The kidney boasts a plethora of homeostatic functions. These include the control of fluid balance, osmolarity and blood pressure, the regulation of electrolyte concentration and acid–base balance, and the elimination of metabolic waste and toxins. The kidneys also play a role in erythrocyte production, via the secretion of erythropoietin. Severe renal disease can therefore result in anaemia because of reduced erythropoietin signalling to the bone marrow. Counterintuitively, some renal conditions (e.g. polycystic kidney disease) can result in polycythaemia. Osteomalacia can develop secondary to chronic renal disease because of the reduction in vitamin D metabolism.

16. D – Apoptosis requires ATP as an energy source
Apoptosis is the process of genetically programmed cell death, which is essential for normal growth and development. It requires ATP, magnesium and calcium-dependent nuclease pathways to allow DNA breakdown at the inter-histone residues. Caspase (cysteine aspartate-specific protease) enzymes are then activated, which ultimately destroy nuclear DNA. Necrosis is another method of cell death, but it is pathological and causes disruption of cellular physiology and results in cell lysis.

17. B – 150 mL
Dead space is the volume of gas within the respiratory system in which gas exchange does not occur. In particular, anatomical dead space refers to the dead space within the conducting zones. In an average adult this is 150 mL. Alveolar dead space is the dead space within the respiratory zone where the alveoli have insufficient blood supply to permit gas exchange. In a non-diseased lung, this is zero.

18. B – Hydrogen ion secretion occurs via H^+-ATPase and Na^+/H^+ co-transporters
Body fluid pH must be maintained within a very narrow range in order to optimize enzymatic function. A small deviation from the normal range can prove life-threatening. The kidneys play a vital role in the

maintenance of acid–base balance. An acid–base disorder can result from respiratory or metabolic means. For example, respiratory failure secondary to chronic obstructive pulmonary disease can lead to impaired ventilation and CO_2 retention. Increased arterial CO_2 acidifies the blood as a result of the Henderson–Hasselbalch equation:

$$pH = pK_a + \log\left(\frac{HCO_3^-}{CO_2}\right)$$

where pK_a = the acid dissociation constant.

Increasing the concentration of CO_2 reduces the HCO_3^-:CO_2 ratio, causing a reduction in pH (i.e. respiratory acidosis). Metabolic acidosis occurs when there is a primary decrease in HCO_3^-. Examples include diabetic ketoacidosis, lactic acidosis and severe diarrhoea. Renal compensation to an acid–base disorder usually takes 2–3 days. The kidneys minimize the pH disturbance in acidosis by increasing acid excretion and HCO_3^- reabsorption. In normal conditions over 99% of the filtered HCO_3^- is reabsorbed, mainly in the proximal tubules. In the proximal tubule, H^+ secretion occurs via Na^+/H^+ countertransport. In the late distal and collecting tubules, H^+ ions are secreted by active transport, i.e. H^+-ATPase. H^+ secretion can be augmented to increase tubular H^+ concentration by as much as 900-fold.

19. E – Younger age of subject
The volume of anatomical dead space increases with age, so the younger the subject, the smaller the volume of dead space. All of the other factors mentioned increase the volume of dead space.

20. C – T-cells with antigen receptors to 'self-antigens' are destroyed by apoptosis in the thymus
Central tolerance is the process by which self-reactive T-cell precursors are destroyed by apoptosis in the thymus so as to prevent autoimmune reactions against self-antigens. The ability of T-lymphocytes to distinguish self from foreign proteins is vital in fighting infection while preventing autoimmune destruction. Self-reactive cells are destroyed by programmed cell death (apoptosis). If tolerance is lost and an immune reaction to host protein develops, autoimmune disease can result. Such conditions often display a genetic trend, and an individual with autoimmune disease will often have more than one condition. Autoimmune diseases include rheumatoid arthritis, vitiligo, type I diabetes mellitus, Addison disease and pernicious anaemia.

21. E – There is a small deoxygenated blood supply in close relation to the gas permeable surface
For optimal gas exchange, a large deoxygenated blood supply is needed in close apposition to the gas permeable surface to maintain an optimal diffusion gradient. Gas exchange takes place primarily at the alveolar surface.

It is associated with maintenance of the acid–base balance. The process of gas exchange is fundamentally dependent on the difference between atmospheric pressure and the pressure within the lungs themselves.

22. B – 500 mL
The tidal volume is the amount of air that is breathed in or out during normal respiration, when the subject is at rest. In the average healthy individual, this is about 0.5 L.

23. D – Portal vein
The portal vein is formed by the confluence of the splenic and inferior mesenteric veins. The fledgling portal vein is then joined early in its course by the superior mesenteric vein. The portal vein carries around 75% of the liver's blood supply.

24. E – Total lung capacity is around 4.8 L in the average adult
Total lung capacity, the total volume of air in the lung after maximal inspiration, is around 6 L in the average adult. The vital capacity is 4.8 L. Vital capacity is the volume of air that can be forcibly expelled (maximal expiration) after maximal inspiration. It is thus the volume of air that, at maximal effort, can be moved in and out of the lung under voluntary control. The remaining volume of air is called the residual volume (1.2 L).

25. B – 0.12–0.2 seconds
The normal P–R interval is between 0.12 and 0.2 seconds, which corresponds to 3–5 small squares on an ECG. The QRS complex should be <0.12 seconds, and the QT interval between 0.38 and 0.42 seconds. The P–R interval represents the time taken for atrial and part of the ventricular depolarization to occur. Atrial systole and ventricular filling occur during this time. The QRS complex is extremely important, as this is the time delay created by the atrioventricular node to allow ventricular filling to occur.

26. A – Cystic artery
The cystic artery is the main arterial supply to the gallbladder. It is usually found in Calot's triangle, an anatomical space defined by the cystic duct, the common hepatic duct and the inferior aspect of the liver. Proper isolation and division of the cystic artery is a crucial step in any operation to remove the gallbladder.

27. E – Ventricular repolarization
Ventricular repolarization is represented on an ECG as the T wave. The P wave represents atrial depolarization and the QRS complex ventricular depolarization. Atrial repolarization is not observed on the normal ECG. T waves give us information regarding the physiological status of the heart. They can be pathologically or physiologically inverted. Pathologically inverted T waves may represent ischaemia or ventricular hypertrophy. It can be normal to have inverted T waves in leads III, aVR and V1.

28. E – None of the above

Intrinsic factor is produced by parietal cells in the fundus and body of the stomach. As B_{12} enters the stomach it becomes bound to haptocorrin. This glycoprotein travels to the duodenum where haptocorrin is digested by pancreatic enzymes. B_{12} can then bind to intrinsic factor.

29. C – R wave

The R wave reflects a rapid depolarization down the intraventricular septum towards the cardiac apex just before the division into the left and right bundles divide. The R wave can be particularly informative with regard to the muscle bulk of the myocardium. Hypertrophic hearts have a larger mass and will therefore have a larger electrical complex. It is important to take the size of the R wave in the context of the patient. For example, a young, slim patient may have large complexes on ECG but a normal echo. This is due to a reduced thoracic impedance.

30. B – Atrial fibrillation with globally small complexes

This patient clearly suffers with chronic obstructive pulmonary disease, and has what is likely an infective exacerbation. Her chest pain is thus related to infection, and further history would likely reveal a pleuritic nature. Infection is a relatively common cause of atrial fibrillation. The reason the complexes are small is due to an increased thoracic impedance from emphysematous lungs. Other causes of increased thoracic impedance include obesity, pleural effusion and pericardial effusion. $S_IQ_{III}T_{III}$ is the textbook finding in pulmonary embolus (S wave in lead I, Q wave in lead II, T inversion in lead III), although sinus tachycardia is more commonly observed in clinical practice. Electrical alternans – the alternation of QRS complex amplitude between beats – occurs in cardiac tamponade. The normal JVP, temperature and productive cough would go against this diagnosis.

31. A – Aortic coarctation

This patient has Turner syndrome, which can be associated with aortic coarctation. It is common that patients are found to have a discrepancy in the blood pressure between the arms and legs, with the blood pressure being higher in the arms. Dissection of the thoracic aorta results in a blood pressure difference between the left and right arms. Aortic stenosis and congestive heart failure result in a narrow pulse pressure, while mitral regurgitation usually has little effect on blood pressure.

32. C – Histamine

Enterochromaffin-like cells are exclusively found in the gastric mucosa. They are stimulated by acetylcholine to produce histamine. Histamine and gastrin act together to stimulate gastric acid secretion. The cells are found within the antrum in the lamina propria. Enterochromaffin cells produce and store 90% of the body's store of serotonin. Serotonin activates both secretory and peristaltic reflexes.

33. D – Rib notching

Rib notching refers to an apparent deformation of the inferior and superior rib borders on imaging and occurs as a result of dilated intercostal collaterals (which help blood bypass the coarctation and supply the descending aorta). There is sparing of the first two ribs as the blood supply for these ribs is not derived from the aorta. Rib notching in coarctation is usually apparent after the age of 6–8 years. In this patient we would find an absence of the typical aortic knuckle, and replacement with a double knuckle (made up of the dilated subclavian artery above and the post-stenotic dilatation of the aorta below). Cardiomegaly and pleural effusions would be unlikely unless there is another underlying pathological process.

34. B – Doxazosin

Doxazosin is an α_1-blocker acting directly on adrenergic receptors to reduce vascular tone. They are also used in benign prostatic hypertrophy. NICE guidelines recommend an ACE inhibitor (or an angiotensin receptor blocker if intolerant) for individuals aged under 55 as the first-line treatment of essential hypertension, and a thiazide diuretic or a calcium channel blocker as the first-line for individuals aged 55 or over or black individuals of any age. If further treatment is required, an ACE inhibitor is added (if not already prescribed), or one of the other two drug types mentioned above. Only when a patient is already on an ACE inhibitor, thiazide and a calcium channel blocker (or has failed trials of these drugs) should fourth-line drugs like alpha-blockers, beta-blockers or further diuretic therapy be added in. Methyldopa stimulates α_2-receptors in the medulla in order to reduce sympathetic outflow. Minoxidil is a K^+ channel activator which is effective in resistant hypertension when combined with a loop diuretic and beta blocker.

35. B – Artery

Loss of elasticity giving rise to a loss of compliance in the larger arteries can lead to an isolated rise in the systolic blood pressure. The affected arteries cannot expand to accommodate the high blood flow at the end of ventricular contraction. This is usually associated with increasing age. NICE guidance recommends treatment for all patients with BP ≥160/100 mmHg, and the decision to treat for those with BP ≥140/90 mmHg is dependent on end organ damage, the presence of diabetes mellitus and the risk of coronary events.

36. E – Tirofiban

Platelet aggregation is thought to begin with an injury to a vessel wall exposing thrombogenic vessel wall collagen, to which platelets directly adhere. Activation of adherent platelets leads to synthesis of a number of chemical mediators – crucial among these is arachidonic acid and thromboxane A2. Aspirin acts here as an irreversible inhibitor of cyclooxygenase, and thus an inhibitor of arachidonic acid and thromboxane A2 synthesis. Crucially, inhibition of cyclooxygenases in the vascular endothelium would lead to a pro-coagulant effect but as these cells, unlike platelets, are nucleated, cyclooxygenase can be regenerated. Thromboxane A2 leads to platelet expression of glycoprotein (GP) IIb/IIIa receptors, subsequent binding of fibrinogen and platelet aggregation. The expression of GPIIb/IIIa receptors is ADP-dependent and thus their expression can be inhibited by the ADP receptor antagonist clopidogrel or adenosine re-uptake inhibitors such as dipyridamole. GPIIb/IIIa antagonists, like tirofiban, act subsequent to GPIIb/IIIa expression to inhibit platelet aggregation. Parenteral prostacyclins suppress the action of mediators like thromboxane A2.

37. D – Popliteal
The popliteal artery is a continuation of the femoral artery and subsequently gives rise to the anterior and posterior tibial arteries. It is palpable in the popliteal fossa. There is a clinical association between aortic aneurysms and popliteal aneurysms, and so if a popliteal artery is felt to be aneurismal, examination of the abdomen is indicated.

38. C – Hyoscine
Hyoscine is an antispasmodic and is often used to relieve colicky abdominal pain. However, it is contraindicated in paralytic ileus, glaucoma and in patients with myasthenia gravis. Side-effects include dry mouth, constipation and urinary retention.

39. E – Superior gluteal artery
The superior gluteal artery is a branch of the internal iliac artery. The internal pudendal artery is a branch of the internal iliac artery that supplies blood to the external genitalia.

40. C – 150 mL
Cerebrospinal fluid lies in the subarachnoid space. The total volume is approximately 130–150 mL. This volume is split between the ventricles of the brain (50 mL) and the spinal cord (100 mL).

41. D – Located in the pons anterior to the cerebellum
The fourth ventricle is one of the cerebrospinal fluid (CSF)-filled cavities within the brain. It is situated in the pons/upper medulla anterior to the cerebellum. It receives CSF from the third ventricle via the cerebral aqueduct in the midbrain. The fourth ventricle drains into the subarachnoid space via the *m*edial foramen of *M*agendie (M for medial and Magendie) and the two *l*ateral foramina of *L*uschka (L for lateral and Luschka).

42. D – Increases by 30–40%
Pregnancy is associated with a number of dramatic physiological changes. In the first trimester, cardiac output increases by 30–40%. This steady rise

can be demonstrated on Doppler echocardiography, as well as up to a 15% increase in heart rate. There is also a steady reduction in systemic vascular resistance.

43. E – Ventricular septal defect

Ventricular septal defects (VSDs) occur in 2 per 1000 births. They can either occur in isolation or as part of a more complex lesion in combination with other congenital cardiac defects. A pansystolic murmur at the left sternal edge may be heard. The size of the VSD has a bearing on the presentation of symptoms. Large VSDs can result in heart failure in infancy with tachypnoea, failure to thrive, feeding difficulties, hepatomegaly and intercostal recession. Spontaneous closure occurs in 30–50% of VSDs.

44. B – Choroid plexus

Cerebrospinal fluid (CSF) is found in the subarachnoid space. It is produced in the choroid plexus of the lateral, third and fourth ventricles. It flows through the ventricles of the brain and passes from the fourth ventricle into the subarachnoid space via the two lateral foramina of Luschka and the medial foramen of Magendie.

45. C – Enlarged left atrium

A left atrial size greater than 5 cm^2 makes DC (direct current) cardioversion extremely difficult. Mitral stenosis can result in an extremely enlarged left atrium, making DC cardioversion almost impossible. Atrial flutter is a macro re-entry circuit and is easily terminated by DC cardioversion. Patients with underlying infection should generally have rate control and treatment of the underlying cause. Young patients with alcohol-induced atrial fibrillation (AF) are often candidates for the 'pill in pocket' regimen (where a single oral dose of an anti-arrhythmic can be taken by a patient at the time and place of onset of AF).

46. C – Depolarization at the bundle of His

The Q wave on an ECG should be relatively small (unless it is pathological), as the muscle bulk is small. It is representative of depolarization at the bundle of His. A so-called 'pathological Q wave' occurs in full thickness (transmural) myocardial infarcts. The result of the full thickness infarct is a non-conducting 'window' of myocardium with no electrical activity. The Q wave is essentially looking through this window at the depolarization occurring on the other side of the heart.

47. A – Arachnoid villi

Cerebrospinal fluid is absorbed by the arachnoid villi into the venous circulation. These are finger-like projections into the subarachnoid space. Obstruction of CSF flow can result in hydrocephalus.

48. D – CN V

The trigeminal nerve (CN V) is responsible for facial sensation. It has three divisions: ophthalmic, maxillary and mandibular. The upper sensory border of the trigeminal nerve is between the ear and skull vertex. The lower sensory border is above the angle of the jaw.

49. A – Ileocolic artery

The ileocolic artery is the lowest of the three colic arteries arising from the superior mesenteric artery. It gives off the appendiceal artery which is ligated during appendectomy.

50. D – Necrosis is accidental cell death which results in the swelling of cells and organelles, and ultimately cell lysis

Necrosis is a pathological process that results in uncontrolled cell death caused by an extrinsic stimulus. It can be induced by acute injury, hypoxia, viruses or drugs and results in swelling of the cell and its organelles, vacuolization and lysis. Macrophages phagocytose the debris, which in turn initiates an inflammatory response. Necrosis must be differentiated from apoptosis. Apoptosis is a function of normal health and development whereby cell death occurs in a regulated and controlled manner.

Questions Paper 10

1. The dorsal column–medial lemniscus pathway transmits which sensory information?
   A. Crude touch
   B. Itch
   C. Pain
   D. Proprioception
   E. Temperature

2. The subarachnoid space ends at which level?
   A. C1
   B. L4
   C. S2
   D. T1
   E. T11

3. Which of the following does the nasal mucosa include?
   A. Lamina propria
   B. Pseudostratified ciliated columnar epithelium
   C. Seromucous glands
   D. Vascular plexus
   E. All of the above

4. Which of the tonsils is lined with ciliated pseudostratified columnar epithelium?
   A. Lingual tonsil
   B. Palatine tonsil
   C. Pharyngeal tonsil
   D. Tubal tonsil
   E. None of the above

5. To which dermatomal level does the nipple correspond?
   A. C8
   B. T1
   C. T2
   D. T3
   E. T4

6. Which one of the following statements about renin is correct?
   A. Increased absorption of Na^+ and Cl^- increases renin secretion.
   B. Renin is a steroid hormone.

C. Renin is secreted by the macula densa within the juxtaglomerular apparatus.
D. The rate of renin secretion is decreased in response to increased renal arterial blood pressure.
E. The rate of renin secretion is increased by parasympathetic stimulation of renal nerves.

7. Which of the following statements regarding refeeding syndrome is *not* correct?
   A. Alcoholic patients and those with malignancy are among those at high risk of developing the syndrome.
   B. Clinical features include rhabdomyolysis, arrhythmias and respiratory and cardiac failure.
   C. Clinical features occur at serum phosphate levels of less than 0.5 mmol/L.
   D. It can be prevented by low caloric introduction of feeds.
   E. Refeeding syndrome is not seen when the patient is fed via parenteral nutrition.

8. With reference to the corticospinal tract, what percentage of fibres do not decussate and descend in the ipsilateral tract?
   A. 5%
   B. 10%
   C. 15%
   D. 20%
   E. 25%

9. Which one of the following is lined with stratified columnar epithelium?
   A. Blood vessels
   B. Ducts of the submandibular glands
   C. Large intestine
   D. Oesophagus
   E. Small intestine

10. Which of the following statements is *not* true in relation to epithelial tissue?
    A. Epithelial cells are attached to one another.
    B. Epithelial cells are separated from the underlying tissue by a basement membrane.
    C. Epithelial tissue covers surfaces with an uninterrupted layer of cells.
    D. Epithelial tissue is non-polarized.
    E. The intracellular space between epithelial cells is small.

11. Which one of the following is lined with stratified keratinized squamous epithelium?
    A. Anus below Hilton's white line
    B. Bladder
    C. Blood vessels

D. Ducts of the submandibular glands

E. Oesophagus

12. Which of the following statements about action potentials is *not* correct?
    A. Action potentials are caused by a sudden opening of voltage gated Na$^+$ channels.
    B. Action potentials are unidirectional.
    C. Action potentials obey the 'all-or-nothing' response.
    D. Action potentials require a threshold potential to be reached before initiation.
    E. The strength of impulse gradually diminishes as the potential travels further from the source of initiation.

13. The respiratory segment of the nasal cavity is lined with which epithelium?
    A. Ciliated pseudostratified columnar
    B. Ciliated stratified columnar
    C. Simple columnar
    D. Simple squamous
    E. Stratified squamous

14. Which extraocular muscle is supplied by the trochlear nerve?
    A. Inferior oblique
    B. Lateral rectus
    C. Medial rectus
    D. Superior oblique
    E. Superior rectus

15. Which cranial nerve is primarily responsible for eye abduction?
    A. Abducens nerve
    B. Facial nerve
    C. Oculomotor nerve
    D. Optic nerve
    E. Trigeminal nerve

16. What movements of the larynx do the cricothyroid muscles produce?
    A. They abduct and externally rotate the arytenoid cartilages which abduct the vocal folds.
    B. They adduct and internally rotate the arytenoid cartilages which adduct the vocal folds.
    C. They lengthen and stretch the vocal folds.
    D. They narrow the laryngeal inlet by decreasing the distance between the arytenoid cartilages and the epiglottis.
    E. None of the above.

17. Osmolality of the extracellular fluid is affected by a number of components. Which one of these does *not* significantly contribute to osmolality?
    A. Glucose
    B. K$^+$

C. Na⁺

   D. Plasma proteins
   E. Urea

18. Which of the turbinates (nasal conchae) are the largest?
    A. Inferior turbinates
    B. Middle turbinates
    C. Outer turbinates
    D. Superior turbinates
    E. None of the above

19. Which one of the following is lined with stratified non-keratinized squamous epithelium?
    A. Anus below Hilton's white line
    B. Bladder
    C. Blood vessels
    D. Ducts of the submandibular glands
    E. Oesophagus

20. Which cranial nerve innervates all three nasal turbinates?
    A. I
    B. II
    C. V
    D. VII
    E. VIII

21. Which of the following is always patent?
    A. Laryngopharynx
    B. Nasopharynx
    C. Oropharynx
    D. All of the above
    E. None of the above

22. Why are action potentials unidirectional within neurons?
    A. Axonal propagation of electrical activity can only occur in one direction.
    B. Consumption of adenosine triphosphate prevents bidirectional propagation.
    C. Na⁺ channels behind the action potential become refractory, and so are unable to depolarize again immediately.
    D. Na⁺ ions travel down their concentration gradient along the axon.
    E. Recruited voltage-gated Ca²⁺ channels open more slowly, preventing reversed depolarization.

23. Which one of the following nerve fibre types is *not* myelinated?
    A. Type A alpha
    B. Type A delta
    C. Type A gamma

D. Type B

E. Type C

24. From which of the following is the epidermis derived?

    A. Ectoderm

    B. Endoderm

    C. Mesoderm

    D. All of the above

    E. None of the above

25. Which is the largest of the paranasal sinuses?

    A. Ethmoid air cells

    B. Frontal sinus

    C. Maxillary sinus

    D. Sphenoidal sinus

    E. None of the above

26. Which of the following correctly describes the series of events that make up the reflex arc of a knee jerk?

    A. Stretch of tendon and muscle; detected by afferent sensory neuron within muscle spindle; synapse with interneuron in dorsal root ganglion; synapse with motor neuron in ventral horn; motor efferent to muscle end plate; contraction of muscle

    B. Stretch of tendon and muscle; detected by afferent sensory neuron within muscle spindle; synapse with motor neuron in dorsal horn; motor efferent to motor end plate; contraction of muscle.

    C. Stretch of tendon and muscle; detected by afferent sensory neuron within muscle spindle; synapse with motor neuron in dorsal root ganglion; motor efferent to motor end plate; contraction of muscle

    D. Stretch of tendon and muscle; detected by efferent sensory neuron within muscle spindle; synapse with motor neuron in ventral horn; motor afferent to motor end plate; contraction of muscle

    E. Stretch of tendon and muscle; detected by afferent sensory neuron within muscle spindle; synapse with motor neuron in ventral horn; motor efferent to muscle end plate; contraction of muscle

27. Which one of the following neurotransmitters is released at the synaptic junctions of motor fibres?

    A. Acetylcholine

    B. Glutamate

    C. Noradrenaline

    D. Serotonin

    E. Substance P

28. Which is the only laryngeal muscle innervated by the external branch of the superior laryngeal nerve?

    A. Cricothyroid

    B. Lateral cricoarytenoid

C. Posterior cricoarytenoid
D. Sternothyroid
E. Thyroarytenoid

29. Which cells are responsible for maintaining the clarity of the cornea?
   A. Columnar cells
   B. Cones
   C. Endothelial cells
   D. Epithelial cells
   E. Squamous cells

30. The superior and recurrent laryngeal nerves are branches of which cranial nerve?
   A. VII
   B. IX
   C. X
   D. XI
   E. XII

31. Which one of the following statements about acetylcholine (ACh) is correct?
   A. ACh binds solely with nicotinic receptors.
   B. ACh is synthesized from tyrosine.
   C. ACh is the principal excitatory neurotransmitter within the central nervous system.
   D. Acetylcholinesterase catalyses the breakdown of ACh into choline and acetyl-CoA.
   E. Myasthenia gravis describes a disease in which antibodies are formed against ACh receptors at the neuromuscular junction.

32. An elderly patient is found to be hyponatraemic. Which of the following tests would you request next?
   A. Chest X-ray
   B. Plasma osmolality, urinary sodium and osmolality
   C. Short synacthen test
   D. Thyroid function tests
   E. Urgent ECG

33. What does troponin T bind to?
   A. Actin
   B. Actinin
   C. Calcium
   D. Myosin
   E. Tropomyosin

34. Which one of the following acts to inhibit the secretion of vasopressin?
   A. Alcohol
   B. Angiotensin II

C. MDMA
D. Nausea
E. Stress, including pain

35. What is the major risk of rapidly rehydrating a patient following prolonged dehydration?
A. Cerebral oedema
B. Excessive loss of electrolytes via the urine
C. Hyperkalaemia
D. Pulmonary oedema
E. Refeeding syndrome

36. Which one of the following statements is true about cells within the nervous system?
A. Degeneration of axons cannot occur after birth.
B. Motor fibres have their cell bodies within dorsal root ganglia.
C. Sensory fibres have their cell bodies within the ventral horn or the brain.
D. The endoneurium is made up of myelin.
E. They are derived from the ectoderm.

37. Local anaesthetics block the sensation of pain. Which one of the following is true regarding their mechanism of action?
A. They inhibit the Na^+/K^+ ATPase pump.
B. They inhibit the opening of voltage-gated Na^+ channels.
C. They reduce the threshold potential for action potential generation.
D. They stimulate the Na^+/K^+ ATPase pump.
E. They stimulate the opening of voltage-gated K^+ channels.

38. Which of the following statements regarding Na^+ homeostasis is *not* correct?
A. Aldosterone increases Na^+–K^+ ATPase activity within principal cells, but has no effect upon epithelial Na^+ channels.
B. Almost all Na^+ excretion occurs within the kidney.
C. Na^+ excretion is dependent upon extracellular fluid volume and osmolality because Na^+ concentration is the main determining factor for both of these.
D. Reabsorption of Na^+ occurs throughout the whole renal tubule, but is most important within principal cells.
E. The need for Na^+ excretion is primarily detected via stretch receptors, receptors within the hypothalamus and macula densa, and the baroreceptors.

39. Which of the following is *not* a cause of increased interstitial fluid volume?
A. Decreased plasma protein levels
B. Increased capillary permeability caused, for example, by histamine, substance P and kinins

C. Increased precapillary constriction
D. Prolonged standing
E. Retention of Na⁺ and water within extracellular fluid

40. Which cells are responsible for the smooth and regular surface of the cornea?
    A. Columnar cells
    B. Cones
    C. Endothelial cells
    D. Epithelial cells
    E. Squamous cells

41. Which cranial nerve supplies the upper lid of the eye?
    A. Abducens nerve
    B. Facial nerve
    C. Oculomotor nerve
    D. Optic nerve
    E. Trigeminal nerve

42. Which of the following combinations of symptoms and signs could be consistent with aspirin overdose?
    A. Respiratory depression, otalgia, headache, nausea and vomiting, renal failure
    B. Respiratory depression, pinpoint pupils, drowsiness and reduced Glasgow coma score
    C. Tinnitus, respiratory depression, respiratory acidosis, vertigo, hyperthermia
    D. Tinnitus, vertigo, arrhythmias, hyperventilation, respiratory alkalosis, hyperthermia
    E. Tinnitus, vertigo, hyperventilation, nausea and vomiting, metabolic acidosis, respiratory alkalosis

43. A 36-year-old woman has rheumatoid arthritis and has been on methotrexate for the past 3 months. Her joint pain and inflammation have worsened over the past few weeks and her rheumatologist prescribed ibuprofen and omeprazole 10 days ago. She visits her GP, as her pain has largely responded but her joint inflammation remains unchanged. What is the most appropriate course of action?
    A. Keep her on her current medication and review in 2 weeks' time
    B. Refer her to a different rheumatologist for a second opinion
    C. Stop omeprazole but continue ibuprofen
    D. Switch ibuprofen to an alternative NSAID and continue with omeprazole
    E. Switch ibuprofen to paracetamol and continue omeprazole

44. A 40-year-old woman has been regularly taking a non-steroidal anti-inflammatory drug (NSAID) for the past 6 weeks and has been experiencing diarrhoea, tiredness and shortness of breath during exertion.

Her full blood count showed haemoglobin 8.2 g/dL and mean cell volume 104 fL. A blood film showed reticulocytes and spherocytes. Which NSAID is most likely responsible for these side-effects?
A. Celecoxib
B. Fenbufen
C. Mefenamic acid
D. Piroxicam
E. Rofecoxib

45. Patients with asplenia are susceptible to which of the following pathogens?
A. *Candida albicans, Entamoeba histolytica, Aspergillus flavus*
B. *Candida albicans, Haemophilus influenzae, Mycoplasma pneumoniae*
C. *Chlamydia trachomatis, Yersinia enterocolitica, Salmonella typhi*
D. *Haemophilus influenzae, Neisseria meningitidis, Streptococcus pneumoniae*
E. *Neisseria meningitidis, Mycoplasma pneumoniae, Chlamydia pneumoniae*

46. Select the clinical scenario which is most likely to be the result of lymphatic system disease.
A. A 7-year-old boy presents with right knee swelling, pain and a fever and is limping.
B. A 19-year-old woman presents with lip and tongue swelling, a new itchy rash and is short of breath after ingesting peanuts.
C. A 20-year-old man presents with a swollen, tender, hot left leg two days after flying home from Australia.
D. A 47-year-old woman with known breast cancer presents with acute-onset right arm swelling. The arm is not hot or tender.
E. A 79-year-old woman fell onto her outstretched right hand and now has a swollen tender right wrist.

47. Which common complication may result from radioiodine treatment in hyperthyroidism?
A. Agranulocytosis
B. Goitre
C. Hypothyroidism
D. Myxoedema coma
E. Thyroid storm

48. What does troponin C bind to?
A. Actin
B. Actinin
C. Calcium
D. Myosin
E. Tropomyosin

49. What is the membrane potential of skeletal muscle?
    A. −80 mV
    B. +80 mV
    C. −90 mV
    D. +90 mV
    E. + 95 mV

50. What is the name of the five-carbon compound that is found in the tricyclic acid cycle?
    A. Acetyl-CoA
    B. Citrate
    C. Oxaloacetate
    D. Oxoglutarate
    E. Succinate

Answers Paper 10

1. D – Proprioception

The dorsal column–medial lemniscus pathway transmits fine touch, vibration and proprioceptive information. The spinothalamic tract transmits information about pain, temperature, itch and crude touch.

2. C – S2

The subarachnoid space extends from the basal cisterns surrounding the brainstem superiorly to the level of S2. It is the space between the arachnoid membrane and pia mater which is filled with cerebrospinal fluid and contains the large blood vessels that supply the brain and spinal cord.

3. E – All of the above

The nasal passages contain the cells which are able to condition air before it reaches the more delicate alveolar tissue. Each has a different function. The ciliated epithelium expels irritants, the seromucous glands provide mucous and the vascular plexus allows for humidification and warming of the inhaled air.

4. C – Pharyngeal tonsil

The pharyngeal tonsils (adenoids), which are located in the roof of the pharynx, are lined with respiratory epithelium, and because of this they also lack crypts. They are a mass of lymphoid tissue situated at the very back of the nose. Other tonsils are usually lined with non-keratinized stratified squamous epithelium.

5. E – T4

The nipple corresponds to the level of the T4 dermatome. A dermatome is an area of skin which is supplied by a single spinal nerve. Identifying specific dermatomes is important when assessing spinal trauma and specific landmarks such as the nipple (mostly helpful in the males) aid in determining levels of pathology.

6. D – The rate of renin secretion is decreased in response to increased renal arterial blood pressure

The juxtaglomerular apparatus is composed of (1) the macula densa and (2) granular cells within the wall of the afferent arteriole. Renin, a protease enzyme, is secreted by the granular cells. Secretion of renin is increased by sympathetic stimulation via renal nerves, circulating catecholamines and prostaglandins. Renin secretion is inhibited by increased afferent arteriolar pressure, angiotensin II, vasopressin and the absorption of

Na⁺ and Cl⁻. The concentration of NaCl within the blood is sensed by the macula densa.

7. E – Refeeding syndrome is not seen when the patient is fed via parenteral nutrition
Refeeding syndrome describes the characteristic morbidity and mortality that can arise from changes in metabolism caused by feeding after prolonged starvation. During periods of starvation, carbohydrate intake is reduced and therefore insulin secretion is also reduced. The metabolism of fat and protein during this time to produce energy depletes intracellular phosphate and other electrolytes. When eating recommences, insulin secretion is stimulated again and results in an increased uptake of phosphate by cells. This results in a markedly reduced serum phosphate level. Both parenteral and enteral routes of feeding can cause refeeding syndrome.

8. A – 5%
About 5% of fibres remain uncrossed and descend in the ipsilateral corticospinal tract. At the pyramidal decussation, 80% of the fibres pass in the lateral corticospinal tract and about 15% in the anterior corticospinal tract.

9. B – Ducts of the submandibular glands
The ducts of the submandibular glands are lined with stratified columnar epithelium. Columnar cells line the apical layer and the lower cells are cuboidal. They become stratified as they approach the opening into the oral cavity.

10. D – Epithelial tissue is non-polarized
Epithelial cells differ from connective tissue by being polarized. Their apical surface is exposed and the basal surface lies on the underlying connective tissue. Polarization allows the cells to maintain a specific arrangement with respect to their intracellular organelles and the consequent directional transport of materials.

11. A – Anus below Hilton's white line
Hilton's white line is the boundary within the anal canal below which the lymphatics drain to the superficial inguinal nodes. This line represents the transition between non-keratinized stratified squamous epithelium (above) and keratinized stratified squamous epithelium (below). The keratinized squamous epithelium is important in areas of constant abrasion as the cells can be replaced before the basement membrane is exposed. Keratinization allows the layer to be kept hydrated.

12. E – The strength of impulse gradually diminishes as the potential travels further from the source of initiation
The initiation of an action potential is dependent upon the opening of voltage gated (or sensitive) sodium ion (Na⁺) channels. These channels

are voltage gated, so that they will only open when the optimal threshold of electrical balance has been reached, a membrane potential of around −55 mV. Once this potential is reached however, their opening creates a rapid influx of Na^+ ions into the neuronal cell, resulting in a rapid depolarization. The all-or-nothing response refers to the fact that a smaller change in membrane potential below the threshold will not initiate a response, but once the threshold is reached, it initiates a standard 'one-size-fits-all' strength of response that propagates along the axon in one direction only and remains consistent in its impulse strength irrespective of how far the impulse travels.

13. A – Ciliated pseudostratified columnar
The respiratory segment is lined with ciliated pseudostratified columnar epithelium. This is in contrast to the olfactory segment which is lined with non-ciliated pseudostratified columnar epithelium.

14. D – Superior oblique
The trochlear nerve is the fourth cranial nerve and supplies the superior oblique muscle, thus causing intorsion (internal rotation), depression and abduction of the eye. The trochlear nerve leaves the brain stem via the dorsal aspect and it decussates before reaching its target muscle. The fourth nerve is rarely impaired on its own, but if it is, it is normally secondary to trauma.

15. A – Abducens nerve
The abducens nerve (CN VI) supplies the lateral rectus, which causes the eye to abduct. Abduction describes the movement of the eye away from the median (saggital) plane of the body. A sixth nerve palsy is implicated in much pathology including multiple sclerosis, a pontine stroke and Wernicke encephalopathy, and it can be a false localizing sign with increased intracranial pressure.

16. C – They lengthen and stretch the vocal folds
The cricothyroid muscles are able to lengthen and stretch the vocal folds by tilting the thyroid cartilage lamina backwards. This leads to higher pitch phonation. It is the only laryngeal muscle innervated by the external branch of the superior laryngeal nerve.

17. B – K^+
The main factors determining plasma and extracellular osmolality are the concentrations of Na^+, urea and glucose. Plasma proteins make only a small contribution, and K^+, because it is predominantly intracellular, has no appreciable contribution. If there is an increase in extracellular fluid, osmolality occurs as a result of a solute such as urea, because this diffuses readily across cell membranes (in comparison to Na^+). The intracellular fluid osmolality will also increase, and osmoreceptors will not be stimulated.

18. A – Inferior turbinates

The inferior turbinates are the largest. They are mostly involved in humidifying, heating and directing airflow. They extend horizontally along the lateral wall of the nasal cavity and they consist of a lamina of spongy bone.

19. E – Oesophagus

The oesophagus is lined with non-keratinized squamous epithelium, which is important in areas of constant abrasion as the cells can be replaced before the basement membrane is exposed.

20. C – V

All three turbinates are innervated by the fifth (trigeminal) nerve. They convey both pain and temperature sensation. The first cranial nerve (olfactory) innervates primarily the superior turbinate and to some extent the middle turbinates.

21. B – Nasopharynx

The nasopharynx is the uppermost part of the pharynx. It extends from the base of the skull to the upper surface of the soft palate. It always remains patent. Anteriorly it communicates through the choanae with the nasal cavities.

22. C – Na^+ channels behind the action potential become refractory, and so are unable to depolarize again immediately

After the Na^+ channel opens, it rapidly becomes refractory and will not reopen until this refractory period has passed. This ensures that the action potential travels in one direction along the axon. The presence of Na^+ ions within the neuron does result in a more positive charge, and this causes increased opening of the voltage-sensitive Na^+ channels. However, the Na^+ channels do not open as a result of a Na^+ chemical concentration gradient alone. Axons are able to propagate electrical activity in both directions, as is seen with local potentials. Action potential propagation within neurons does not involve Ca^{2+} ion channels, and consumption of ATP does not prevent bidirectional propagation.

23. B – Type A delta

Myelination of nerve fibres allows more rapid conduction of action potential along the fibre. All types of A and B fibres are myelinated, and so are used by nerves relying upon fast conduction of nerve impulses. Type C nerve fibres are unmyelinated, and therefore conduct nerve impulses more slowly.

24. A – Ectoderm

The epidermis is derived from ectoderm. The ectoderm is the outermost germ layer. It is the layer which differentiates to form the nervous system, tooth enamel and also the epidermis. It is composed of three parts: the external ectoderm, the neural crest and the neural tube. The endoderm forms the lining of most of the gastrointestinal tract (except that of the mouth, pharynx and lower rectum which are lined by ectoderm) and other organs. The mesoderm is able to differentiate into a number of different tissues.

25. C – Maxillary sinus
The maxillary sinus is the largest of the paranasal sinuses. They are situated within the maxillary bones under the eyes. All the sinuses are lined with ciliated pseudostratified columnar epithelium.

26. E – Stretch of tendon and muscle; detected by afferent sensory neuron within muscle spindle; synapse with motor neuron in ventral horn; motor efferent to muscle end plate; contraction of muscle
Under normal circumstances, stretching a tendon produces reflex contraction of muscle. The typical spinal reflex arc occurs as follows: the stretch of tendon and muscle is detected by afferent sensory neurons within the muscle spindle; these synapse with motor neurons in the ventral horn, and then with motor efferents to the muscle end plate, resulting in contraction of muscle. If a patient has suffered a stroke or spinal injury proximal to where a reflex is tested, descending inhibition of the spinal reflex occurs, creating brisker reflexes when they are examined.

27. A – Acetylcholine
Acetylcholine binds to muscarinic and nicotinic receptors. Nicotinic receptors are ion-gated channels found within the motor end plate of neuromuscular junctions (NMJs). A propagated action potential arriving at the presynaptic cleft of the NMJ facilitates the release of acetylcholine, which binds to nicotinic receptors, causing a conformational change to open the ion channel. This allows the influx of sodium ions into the postsynaptic cleft and depolarization of T-tubules.

28. A – Cricothyroid
The external branch of the superior laryngeal nerve supplies the cricothyroid muscle. This branch is also susceptible to damage during thyroidectomy as it lies just deep to the superior thyroid artery.

29. C – Endothelial cells
The corneal endothelial cells are low cuboidal or squamous cells which are rich in mitochondria. They are continuously pumping out fluid from the tissue to maintain the clarity of the cornea, helping to prevent subsequent corneal oedema. These cells do not regenerate and instead stretch to compensate for dead cells. This can have an impact on fluid regulation within the cornea and lead to reduced transparency.

30. C – X
Both the superior and recurrent laryngeal nerves are branches of the vagus nerve (cranial nerve X). The laryngeal nerve is the first branch of the vagus nerve, which then divides to form the aforementioned branches which innervate the larynx.

31. E – Myasthenia gravis describes a disease in which antibodies are formed against ACh receptors at the neuromuscular junction

Acetyl-CoA and choline combine to form ACh, however acetylcholinesterase catalyses the breakdown of ACh into choline and acetate. ACh is the neurotransmitter found at the neuromuscular junctions within the skeletal muscle. Glutamate, by contrast, is an important excitatory neurotransmitter within the central nervous system. ACh can bind to either muscarinic or nicotinic receptors. Noradrenaline, not ACh, is formed from tyrosine.

32. A – Chest X-ray

A chest X-ray (to look for a pulmonary cause of inappropriate antidiuretic hormone secretion; e.g. lung cancer, TB, pneumonia), short synacthen test (to exclude Addison disease) or thyroid function tests (to rule out severe hypothyroidism) would all be appropriate tests when investigating hyponatraemia. The most useful initial test, however, is to distinguish whether the low sodium is caused by an increase in sodium excretion or by inappropriate water retention. Comparisons between urinary and plasma sodium and osmolality will help to make these distinctions.

33. E – Tropomyosin

Thin myofilaments contain three different proteins: actin, troponin and tropomyosin. Actin is a long-stranded protein. Two alpha helix strands of actin proteins are twisted around each other to form a double-stranded helix. Twisting around the groove between the two actin alpha helix strands lie two alpha helix strands of tropomyosin, another long-stranded protein. Tropomyosin blocks binding sites of myosin in the actin groove. Along this helical structure, at regular intervals, are troponin molecules. The troponin molecules are attached to both the actin and tropomyosin strands. Troponin is a trimeric protein with three subunits: troponin C binds to Ca^{2+} ions; troponin T binds to tropomyosin; and troponin I binds to actin.

34. A – Alcohol

Alcohol has an inhibitory effect on vasopressin secretion, explaining the increased need to micturate and the possibility of dehydration upon consumption. Angiotensin II released in response to hypovolaemia helps to stimulate fluid retention via vasopressin release. Increased secretion of vasopressin and fluid retention is often seen in patients post surgery as a result of a stress response. Nausea and ingestion of MDMA also stimulate vasopressin secretion.

35. A – Cerebral oedema

During periods of dehydration, the brain synthesizes osmolytes. Cerebral oedema can complicate rapid rehydration, because the intracellular concentration of osmolytes has become abnormally high and thus encourages excessive movement of water into cells. Refeeding syndrome describes the phenomenon encountered in malnourished patients when fat metabolism is rapidly converted to carbohydrate metabolism. Increased secretion of insulin causes rapid cellular uptake of phosphate, resulting in severe hypophosphataemia. The consequences of severe hypophosphataemia include rhabdomyolysis, acute haemolytic anaemia and fatal arrhythmias.

36. E – They are derived from the ectoderm
The entire nervous system is of ectodermal origin. Peripheral nerve axons can regenerate, but regeneration of axons is limited within the central nervous system. Sensory fibres have their cell bodies within dorsal root ganglia or the brain, and motor fibre cell bodies are located within the ventral horn of the spinal cord. Sensory and motor nerves travel together within a peripheral nerve. These are wrapped within a connective tissue sheath, called an endoneurium.

37. B – They inhibit the opening of voltage-gated Na^+ channels
Local anaesthetics inhibit voltage-gated Na^+ channels and therefore the generation of action potentials at the axon hillock. Type C fibres are most sensitive to local anaesthetics. Reducing the threshold potential would increase action potential generation, as would inhibiting the Na^+/K^+ ATPase pump. Local anaesthetics do not stimulate the Na^+/K^+ ATPase pump or opening of the K^+ channels.

38. A – Aldosterone increases Na^+–K^+ ATPase activity within principal cells, but has no effect upon epithelial Na^+ channels
Because Na^+ is the predominant extracellular fluid (ECF) cation, its concentration within the ECF has the greatest influence upon ECF volume, osmolality and Na^+ excretion. Around 90–95% of Na^+ excretion occurs within the kidney. Epithelial Na^+ channels within principal cells are the most important site of Na^+ reabsorption within the kidney, although reabsorption does occur throughout the renal tubules. Aldosterone increases both Na^+–K^+ ATPase activity and epithelial Na^+ channel efficiency.

39. C – Increased precapillary constriction
Oedema is the accumulation of abnormally large volumes of interstitial fluid. Retention of Na^+ and H_2O within the extracellular fluid results in an increased volume of both intravascular and interstitial fluid. Plasma proteins exert an oncotic force that retains fluid within the intravascular space. If levels of these proteins fall, fluid can more readily move into the interstitial space and is not as readily reabsorbed within the postcapillary bed. Increased capillary permeability also causes increased loss of plasma proteins, which is followed by a movement of a fluid into the interstitium. Increased postcapillary constriction will create an increased hydrostatic pressure, which may overcome the oncotic pressure and force fluid out into the interstitial space. During movement, skeletal muscle-induced contraction of veins helps to keep venous pressure low and thereby helps

the return of fluid into veins. If an individual stands for long periods, this increases venous pressure, therefore making fluid accumulation within the interstitium more likely.

40. D – Epithelial cells

The anterior surface of the cornea is lined with non-keratinized stratified squamous epithelium that readily regenerates. This, with the addition of the tear film, provides a smooth and regular surface for the cornea to refract light. If there is irregularity or oedema of the epithelial layer there is disruption of the air–tear interface which will consequently lead to reduced visual acuity.

41. C – Oculomotor nerve

The oculomotor nerve (CN III) supplies all the extraocular muscles: superior rectus, inferior rectus, medial rectus and inferior oblique muscles. The two outstanding extraocular muscles, the lateral rectus and superior oblique, are supplied by the abducens (CN VI) and trochlear nerve (CN IV), respectively. The oculomotor nerve also supplies the levator palpebrae superioris muscle (controls the upper eye lid) and causes pupil constriction. A third nerve palsy therefore leads to ptosis, a large pupil and an eye that is deviated 'down and out' (infraducted and abducted).

42. E – Tinnitus, vertigo, hyperventilation, nausea and vomiting, metabolic acidosis, respiratory alkalosis

Because of its mechanism of action in inhibiting cyclooxygenase-1 and 2, aspirin is pharmacologically considered a non-steroidal anti-inflammatory drug (NSAID), although it is also classed as a salicylate. In overdose the characteristic signs and symptoms it produces are different from those of an overdose of other NSAIDs. Aspirin overdose has three major groups of effects: (1) middle ear damage, causing tinnitus, vertigo and associated nausea and vomiting; (2) respiratory centre stimulation, causing hyperventilation and a resultant respiratory alkalosis; and (3) uncoupling of oxidative phosphorylation, causing hyperthermia and metabolic acidosis.

43. A – Keep her on her current medication and review in 2 weeks' time

Although the analgesic effect of NSAIDs usually takes around a week to develop, their anti-inflammatory effect can take up to 3 weeks to become clinically apparent. In this scenario, more time should be given before considering changing the patient's current regimen. If there is still no effect after 3–4 weeks of regular ibuprofen use, consider switching to a different NSAID, as individual responses to different NSAIDs are variable and difficult to predict. It may take several months of trying different NSAIDs before the most suitable one for a particular patient is found. Omeprazole as a gastroprotectant against ulceration should be continued. Only after two failed disease-modifying anti-rheumatic drugs (DMARDs) would agents such as anti-tumour necrosis factor monoclonal antibodies be considered. DMARDs should be tried for 6 months before an absence of effect is considered a failure.

44. C – Mefenamic acid

Mefenamic acid can give rise to diarrhoea and can occasionally induce autoimmune haemolytic anaemia. The features of autoimmune haemolytic anaemia are low haemoglobin, macrocytosis (because of compensatory reticulocyte proliferation) and spherocytosis on blood film. The direct antiglobulin test (Coombs test) is positive.

45. D – *Haemophilus influenzae, Neisseria meningitidis, Streptococcus pneumoniae*

Patients who have had a splenectomy, either surgically or an autosplenectomy as a result of vaso-occlusion (for example in patients with sickle cell disease), are at an increased risk of developing overwhelming sepsis from blood-borne infection by encapsulated organisms. This is because the spleen is the key lymphoid organ involved in filtering and trapping blood-borne antigens. Asplenic patients should be on prophylactic daily penicillin, usually for life, and should be vaccinated against these infections.

46. D – A 47-year-old woman with known breast cancer presents with acute-onset right arm swelling. The arm is not hot or tender

This woman has acute onset lymphoedema, most likely as a consequence of breast tumour cells infiltrating the axillary lymphatics and causing occlusion. Accumulated lymph results in swelling. The other clinical scenarios, respectively, represent likely cases of deep vein thrombosis, anaphylaxis, septic arthritis and Colles fracture.

47. C – Hypothyroidism

Radioiodine is an effective treatment for hyperthyroidism. It emits β-particles (high-energy, high-speed electrons) which have a cytotoxic action on thyroid follicular cells. The resulting destruction decreases thyroid hormone secretion and therefore will reduce hormone levels. The common complication is an underactive thyroid gland producing symptoms of hypothyroidism. Thyroid hormone replacement therapy, e.g. levothyroxine, may be commenced if this occurs. This radioiodine-thyroxine treatment sequence is commonly referred to as a type of 'block and replace' regimen.

48. C – Calcium

Thin myofilaments contain three different proteins: actin, troponin and tropomyosin. Actin is a long-stranded protein. Two alpha helix strands of actin proteins are twisted around each other to form a double-stranded helix. Twisting around the groove between the two actin alpha helix strands lie two alpha helix strands of tropomyosin, another long-stranded protein. Tropomyosin blocks binding sites of myosin in the actin groove. Along this helical structure, at regular intervals, are troponin molecules.

The troponin molecules are attached to both the actin and tropomyosin strands. Troponin is a trimeric protein with three subunits: troponin C binds to Ca^{2+} ions; troponin T binds to tropomyosin; and troponin I binds to actin.

49. C - −90 mV

The membrane potential of skeletal muscle is around −90 mV. An action potential is initiated when acetylcholine is released from the motor neuron. An action potential lasts for about 2–4 milliseconds. The contraction of a muscle is triggered via the initiation and propagation of an action potential along the muscle fibre membrane.

50. D – Oxoglutarate

Oxaloacetate is a four-carbon molecule. It reacts with a two-carbon molecule of acetyl-CoA to form the six-carbon compound citrate. At this point in the citric acid cycle one molecule of carbon dioxide is removed to form the five-carbon compound oxoglutarate.

Index

A

A-bands, 35
Abciximab, 51
Abdominal aneurysmal disease, 110
Abducens nerve (CN VI), 191
ABO blood group, 111
ACE inhibitor, *see* Angiotensin-converting enzyme inhibitor
Acetylcholine (ACh) receptors, 16, 19, 194
Acetyl-CoA, 12, 17, 72
Acidaemia, 149
Acoustic neuroma, 75
Actin, 33, 194, 197
Action potential, 190, 198
Activated partial thromboplastin time (APTT), 17
Acute epiglottitis, 129, 134
Acute renal failure, 167
Addison disease, 76
Adductor pollicis brevis, 54
Adenosine diphosphate (ADP), 147
Adenosine monophosphate (AMP), 14
Adenosine triphosphate (ATP), 14, 34, 170
β-Adrenergic receptors, 14
Afferent neuron, 69
Agranulocytosis, 74
Albumins, 96
Alcohol, 194
Aldosterone, 195
Allopurinol, 35, 53
Alpha-motoneurons, 150
Alternative complement pathway, 36
Alveolar development, 133
Amacrine cells, 57
Amino acids, 127
Aminoacyl-tRNA, 91
Aminoglycosides, 72, 74
Amisulpride, 132
Amitriptyline, 19
Amlodipine, 90, 153
AMP, *see* Adenosine monophosphate
Anal canal, 190
Anaphylatoxins, 93
Angiotensin-converting enzyme (ACE) inhibitor, 15, 19, 54, 58, 152, 155
Angiotensinogen, 169
Angiotensin-receptor blocker (ARB), 15, 54
Anion gap, 11
Anterior median fissure, 96
Aortic arch syndrome, 39

Aortic coarctation, 173
APC (adenomatous polyposis coli) tumour suppressor gene, 18, 35, 111
Apoptosis, 17, 19, 170, 177
Appendicular skeleton, 111
APTT, *see* Activated partial thromboplastin time
Arachnoid villi, 176
ARB, *see* Angiotensin-receptor blocker
Arteries, loss of compliance in, 174
Arteriole, 91
Aspirin (acetylsalicylic acid), 90, 174, 196
ATP, *see* Adenosine triphosphate
Atrial fibrillation, 148, 173
Atrioventricular node (AVN), 55
Auerbach's plexus, 14, 112
Autonomic ganglion, 131
Autonomic nervous system, 128, 131
Avascular necrosis, 93
Axon diameter, 35

B

Bacterial cell walls, 36
Bacterial infection, 39
Bacteroides fragilis, 15
Basal ganglia, 11
Basilar artery, 37
Basophils, 94, 96
Bendroflumethiazide, 73, 153
Benign prostatic hyperplasia (BPH), 16
Benzodiazepine, 17, 127, 130
Beta-blockers, 14, 113
Bicarbonate, circulating actual, 155
Bilateral renal artery stenosis, 15
Bilirubin, 12
Bipolar disorder, 73
Bisoprolol, 113, 153
Bladder malignancy, 169
Bladder smooth muscle, 129
Blood, hydrogen ions in, 150
Blood group A, 17
Blood pH, 150
Blurred vision, 18
B-lymphocytes (B-cells), 89
Bone, lamellar structure of, 112
Bone marrow failure, 111
BPH, *see* Benign prostatic hyperplasia
Bradycardia, 111
Bradykinin, 19

BRCA1 (Breast Cancer 1, early onset) tumour suppressor gene, 19
Breast cancer, 197
Brunner glands, 107
Buprenorphine, 112
Burns (multiple), 73

C

Ca^{2+} channels, 37
Cadherins, 53
Calcium, 34, 132
cAMP, *see* Cyclic adenosine monophosphate
Cancellous bone, 108
Cancer, risk of developing, 114
Carbimazole, 13, 74, 130
Carbon dioxide, 71, 94
Carcinoid tumours, 18
Caseous necrosis, 14
Caspase, 170
Catechol-*O*-methyltransferase (COMT), 13
β-Catenin, 111
Cauda equina, 70
CCK, *see* Cholecystokinin
CD4 receptor, 128
Cellular debris, 111
Cellular migration, 37
Central nervous system (CNS), 35, 131
Central tolerance, 171
Cephalic phase, 168
Cerebral oedema, 194
Cerebrospinal fluid (CSF), 175, 176
Cervical nerves, 89
C5 vertebra, 52
CFTR, *see* Cystic fibrosis transmembrane conductance regulator
Chemotaxis, 136, 147
Chest X-ray, 194
Cholecystokinin (CCK), 168
Choroid plexus, 176
Chromatin, peripheral condensation of 15
Chvostek sign, 131
Ciliary ganglion, 133
Ciliated pseudostratified columnar epithelium, 58, 191
Ciprofloxacin, 91, 93
Citrate, 12, 72, 73
CK, *see* Creatine kinase
Classical complement pathway, 89
Class III reactions, 92
Clavulanic acid, 92
Clexane, 58
Clostridium difficile–associated diarrhoea, 75
Clostridium perfringens, 15

Clozapine, 52, 131
CNS, *see* Central nervous system
Coccyx, 70
Cockcroft–Gault formula, 151
Co-codamol, 112
Coeliac ganglion, 13
Collagen synthesis, inhibition of, 149
Colorectal cancer, 18
Columnar epithelium, 153
Complement components, 114
COMT, *see* Catechol-*O*-methyltransferase
Cone types (retina), 56
Conn syndrome, 76
Conus medullaris, 69
Cornea, anterior surface of, 196
Corneal endothelial cells, 193
Co-trimoxazole, 75
Cough, 134
Cranial nerves VII/IX, 134
Creatine kinase (CK), 53
Creatine phosphokinase, 13
Cricothyroid muscles, 191, 193
Cristae, 74
Cryptococcus infections, 14
CSF, *see* Cerebrospinal fluid
C3b, opsonization and, 92
Cyclic adenosine monophosphate (cAMP), 18, 128, 129
Cyclooxygenase (COX), 38, 39, 109
Cyclooxygenase 1 (COX-1), 135
Cystic artery, 172
Cystic fibrosis transmembrane conductance regulator (CFTR), 18
Cystic medial degeneration, 110
Cytoskeleton, 154
Cytosol, 149

D

Daptomycin, 31
Dead space, 170
Dehydration, 167
Depression, 73
de Quervain thyroiditis, 130
Dermatome, 189
Desmosomes, 52, 147
Diabetes, 69, 110
Diabetic ketoacidosis, 11
Diapedesis, 136
Diaphragmatic pleura, 72
Diazepam, 17
Digoxin, 52, 58
Dihydrofolate reductase, 31, 35
Direct reflex, 132
DNA binding domain, 38

DNA gyrase, 32
Dorsal column–medial lemniscus
  pathway, 189
Doxazosin, 174
Duodenum, 107
Dura mater, 72

E

ECF, *see* Extracellular fluid
Ectoderm, 192, 195
Edinger–Westphal nucleus, 11, 13, 132
EGF, *see* Epithelial growth factor
Elastase, 147
Electrical currents, 36
Empty sella syndrome, 12
Endogenous chemicals, 113
Endothelium, 89
Enteric nervous system, 112
Enterochromaffin-like cells, 173
Enterocytes, 151
Enteroendocrine cells, 18
Enzyme inducers, 53
Epidural, 113
Epithelial cadherin (E-cadherin), 55
Epithelial cells, 190
Epithelial growth factor (EGF), 147
Epithelioid cells, 149
Epitope, 56
Erythrocyte sedimentation rate, 128, 150
Erythropoietin, 95
E-selectin, 90
Ethambutol, 92
Exocytosis, 133
External carotid, 33
Extracellular fluid (ECF), 195
Extracellular osmolality, 191
Eye, ciliary muscle of, 13

F

Factor VIII deficiency, 111
Fasciculus gracilis, 71
Fast fibres, 33
Fat transport, 51
Femoral artery, 32, 51
Fentanyl, 54, 110
Fibrin clot, 148
Fibroblast growth factor (FGF), 147
Finasteride, 16
5q (chromosome), 35
Flight-or-fight response, 16, 128
Flumazenil, 17
Fluoroquinolones, 91, 93
Folic acid, 91, 93

G

GALT, *see* Gut-associated lymphoid tissue
Gamma-aminobutyric acid (GABA), 37, 108, 130
Gamma-motoneurons, 149
Gamma tubulin, 74
Gas exchange, 171
Gastric (hydrochloric) acid, 169
Gastric arteries (right and left), 18
Gastric chief cells, 167
Gastric inhibitory polypeptide (GIP), 168
Gastric veins (left and right), 12
Gastrocnemius, 89
Gastrointestinal system, parasympathetic
  innervation of, 134
Genetics (autosomal dominant), 15
Giant cell arthritis, 69
Glomerular filtration rate (GFR), 170
Glossopharyngeal (IX) nerve, 51
Glossopharyngeal parasympathetic neurons,
  132, 134
Gluconeogenesis, 127
Glucuronyl transferase, 12
Gluteus maximus, 55
Glycopeptide antibiotics, 70
Glycoprotein IIb/IIIa receptors, 89
Goblet cells, 154
'Golfer's elbow,' 95
Golgi apparatus, 34
G-protein receptors, 132
Graves disease, 130
GTPase proteins, 76
Guanosine triphosphate (GTP), 70, 109
Gut-associated lymphoid tissue (GALT), 70, 71

H

Haematopoiesis, 110
Haemoglobin, 15, 91, 94
Haemophilia A, 111
Haemophilus influenzae, 128, 134, 197
Haversian canals, 113
HbS, *see* Sickle cell haemoglobin
Hearing loss, asymmetrical, 75
Hemidesmosomes, 52, 147
Henderson–Hasselbalch equation, 151, 171
Heparin, 17
Hepatic vein, 91
Hereditary retinoblastoma, 69
Hereditary spherocytosis, 129
Heschl's convolution, 12
Hilton's white line, anus below, 190
Histamine, 173
HMG-CoA (3-hydroxy-3-methylglutaryl-
  coenzyme A) reductase, 34, 39

Horner's syndrome, 54
Hot potato voice, 135
Hydrogen ion secretion, 170
Hydroxyapatite, 112
Hyoscine, 175
Hyperaldosteronism, 76
Hypercalcaemia, 52
Hypercholesterolaemia, 34
Hyperkalaemia, 76
Hyperthyroidism, 13, 130, 197
Hypertrophic hearts, 173
Hyperventilation, 150
Hypocalcaemia, 131
Hypogastric nerve, 129
Hyponatraemia, 72, 73
Hypothalamic thermostat, 38, 113

I

Ibuprofen, 130
IgA 56
IGF-1, *see* Insulin-like growth factor-1
IgG antibodies, 57, 89, 133
IL-2, *see* Interleukin 2
IL-8, 133
Ileocolic artery, 177
Ileum, 56, 114
Iliopsoas, 96
Imidazobenzodiazepine, 17
Incomitant strabismus, 75
Inferior gluteal nerve, 55
Inferior turbinates, 192
Inferior vena cava (IVC), 92–93
Infliximab, 35
Innate immune response, 170
Insulin-like growth factor-1 (IGF-1), 147
Integrins, 133
Interferon, 150
Interleukin 2 (IL-2), 38
Intermediate filaments, 152
Internal carotid artery, 32
Interosseous membrane, 153
Interstitial fluid, 167
Intraepithelial lymphocytes, 70
Intrinsic factor, 173
Intrinsic renal failure, 167
Iron deficiency, 109
Isocitrate dehydrogenase, 71
Isosorbide mononitrate, 52
IVC, *see* Inferior vena cava

J

Jejunum, 109, 154
Juxtaglomerular apparatus, 189

K

Kappa segment, 55
Keloid formation, 154
Keratinized epithelium, 155
Ketones, 11
Koilonychia, 109
Krebs cycle, 17, 107

L

Labetalol, 151
β-Lactams, 90
Lactate, 148
Lacteals, 51
Laminins, 37
Lateral epicondyle, 95
L-cells, 58
LDLs, *see* Low-density lipoproteins
Leber hereditary optic neuropathy (LHON), 76
Left atrial size, 176
Left gastric vein, 90
Legionella pneumophila, 18
Leukocytes, 96, 132, 133, 136
Leukotriene B4, 133, 135
Lincosamides, 75
Lipopeptide antibiotics, 31
Lisinopril, 155
Lithium, 73
Liver failure, 113
Loop diuretics, 168
Low-density lipoproteins (LDLs), 34
Ludwig angina, 128
Lung segments, 115
Lymphoedema, 197
Lysosomes, 147

M

MAC, *see* Membrane attack complex
Malaria, 17
Male urethra, 94
Malignant hyperpyrexia, 17
MALT, *see* Mucosa-associated lymphoid tissue
Mannose-binding lectin, 91
Marginal artery of Drummond, 57
Mast cells, 94
Matrix metalloproteinases (MMPs), 154
Maxillary sinus, 193
Meckel diverticulum, 56
Medial longitudinal fasciculus, 73
Mefenamic acid, 197
Meissner's plexus, 71, 127
MELD score, 151
Membrane attack complex (MAC), 93

Ménière disease, 76
Mesoderm, tissues derived from, 153
Messenger RNA (mRNA), 147, 154
Metabolic alkalosis, 12
Methicillin-resistant *Staphylococcus aureus*
  (MRSA), 15
Methyldopa, 174
Metoprolol, 113
Microtubules, 69, 132, 152
Midazolam, 127
Misoprostol, 152
Mitochondria, 34, 37, 73
Mitosis, sequence of, 37
MMPs, *see* Matrix metalloproteinases
Monoclonal antibodies, 51, 151
Monocyte, 52
Morphine, 112
MPO, *see* Myeloperoxidase
mRNA, *see* Messenger RNA
MRSA, *see* Methicillin-resistant
  Staphylococcus aureus
Mucosa-associated lymphoid tissue (MALT), 70
Mu receptor, 108
Muscarinic receptors, 128
Muscle breakdown, 127
Muscularis externa, 14, 112
Muscularis mucosa, 127
Myasthenia gravis, 19, 194
Mycobacteria, 92
Mycobacterium tuberculosis, 14
Mycoplasma tuberculosis, 110
Mycotic aneurysms, 39
Myelinated neurons, 35, 192
Myelinated type B fibre, 130
Myeloperoxidase (MPO), 39

N

Na+ channel, 192, 195
NADH, 17, 71
Na+/K+/2Cl− co-transporter, 168
Nasal passages, 189
Nasopharynx, 192
Necrosis, 15, 177
Necrotizing fasciitis, 14, 15
Neisseria meningitidis, 197
Nephrotoxic drugs, 167
Nervous system, parts of, 131
Neural tube defects, 91
Neurological damage, 93
Neuromuscular junction (NMJ), 16, 19, 193
Neutrophils, 114
Nicorandil, 57
Nicotinic receptors, 34, 135
Nipple, 189

Nitric oxide, 129
5-Nitroimidazoles, 32
Non-steroidal anti-inflammatory drugs
  (NSAIDs), 54, 109, 113, 135, 151, 196
Nordazepam, 130

O

Oculomotor nerve (CN III), 11, 196
Oedema, 195
Oesophagus, 71, 192
Olanzapine, 36, 132
Omeprazole, 73, 152
Opiate withdrawal, 112
Opioid receptors, 108
Opsonization, 92
Optic papilla, 56
Osteoblasts, 31
Osteoclasts, 32
Osteoid osteomas, 112
Osteoid production, 31
Osteomalacia, 170
Osteonecrosis, 93
Ovarian cancer, 19
Ovaries, 37, 38
Oxaloacetate, 12, 17, 72, 77, 107, 198
Oxazolidinones, 74
Oxoglutarate dehydrogenase, 70

P

Paneth cells, 53, 155
Paracetamol, 54, 110
Paralytic squint, 75
Parasympathetic innervation (vagus nerve), 15
Parasympathetic system, 129
Parathyroid hormone (PTH), 127
Parietal cells, 169
Parkinson disease, 13
Partial pressure of carbon dioxide, 150
Partial pressure of oxygen (arterial), 150
Patella, 58, 108
Patent ductus arteriosus (PDA), 169
Patient-controlled analgesia (PCA), 112
PDGF, *see* Platelet-derived growth factor
Pectoral muscles, 11
Pelvic floor, muscles of, 95
Penicillins, 74
Pepsinogen, 167
Peptide YY, 58
Peptidoglycans, 36, 70
Peptidyl-tRNA, 72
Perforating canals, 113
Peripheral nervous system (PNS), 35
Peyer's patches, 114

p53 (protein 53) tumour suppressor
   gene, 36, 114
PGE2, *see* Prostaglandin E2
Phagocytosis, 133
Pharyngeal tonsils (adenoids), 189
Pia mater, 70
Pituitary gland, 12
Plasma proteins, 96, 191
Plasminogen, 96
Platelet aggregation, 89, 174
Platelet count range (normal), 109
Platelet-derived growth factor (PDGF), 147
PNS, *see* Peripheral nervous system
Polyarteritis nodosum, 38
Polycystic kidney disease (PKD), 15
Polycythaemia rubra vera, 75
Popliteal artery, 175
Portal vein, 172
Posterior cerebral artery, 37
Postganglionic neurons, 11, 132
Potassium channels, 73
Potassium iodide, 130
Preganglionic neurons, 131, 132, 133
Pregnancy, 152, 175–176
Primary auditory cortex, 12
P–R interval, 172
Proprioception, 189
Propylthiouracil, 13
Prostacyclin production, inhibition of, 131
Prostaglandin E2 (PGE2), 135
Pterygopalatine ganglion, 134
PTH, *see* Parathyroid hormone
Pulmonary artery, 90
Pulseless disease, 39
Pupillary constriction, 54
Pupillary reflex, disruption of, 69
Pyramidal decussation, 96, 190
Pyridostigmine, 16
Pyrogens, 113
Pyruvate, 12, 72, 107

Q

QRS complex, 55, 172
Quetiapine, 132
Quinine, 16
Quinolones, 32
Q wave, 176

R

RAA axis, *see* Renin–angiotensin–
   aldosterone axis
Radioiodine, 74
Ramipril, 54, 153

Ras gene, mutations in, 76
RB1 (retinoblastoma) gene, 69
RCA, *see* Right coronary artery
Reactive oxygen species, 147
Rectus femoris, 33
Refeeding syndrome, 190, 194–195
Remak bundles, 112
Renal arteries, 92
Renal disease, severe, 170
Renal failure, acute, 167
Renin–angiotensin–aldosterone (RAA)
   axis, 169
Renin secretion, 189
Resolution, 38
Respiration, principle muscles of 11
Respiratory alkalosis, 150
Respiratory bronchioles, 96
Resting potential (neuron membrane), 36
Retina, layers of, 57
Reye syndrome, 90
Rheumatoid arthritis, 151
Rhinovirus, 75
Rib notching, 174
Ribosomes, dissociation of, 19
Rifampicin, 32
Right coronary artery (RCA), 168
Risperidone, 131
Rofecoxib, 109
Rotator cuff muscles, 56
Rough endoplasmic reticulum, 34, 154
R wave, 173

S

Sacral area, 95
SAN, *see* Sinoatrial node
Sarcomere, 32
Sartorius muscle, 33
Scar formation, 154
Schwannoma (vestibular nerve), 75
Selective serotonin reuptake inhibitors
   (SSRIs), 52, 56
Self-reactive cells, 171
Sensory receptor, 69
Sepsis, 197
Septic shock, 114
Serratus anterior, 14
17p (chromosome), 36
Sharpey fibres, 112
Shoulder, medial rotation of, 51
Sickle cell haemoglobin (HbS), 107
Simvastatin, 53
Sinoatrial node (SAN), 57, 168
Skeletal muscle, membrane potential of, 198
Slow fibres, 33

Small intestine, mucosa of, 115
Smooth muscle, 58, 74, 129, 147
Sodium channels, 31
S (synthesis) phase (cell cycle), 33
Sphincter relaxation, 134
Spinal reflex, 193
Spleen lymphatics, 55
Splenectomy, 197
Splenic artery, 110
Spongy bone, 108
Squamous cell carcinoma, 52
Squamous epithelium, 152
SSRIs, *see* Selective serotonin
        reuptake inhibitors
Staphylococcus aureus, 110, 133
Statins, 34, 39, 53
Steroid receptor, 38
Stomach, 71, 147, 155
Stratified squamous epithelium, 71
Streptococcus, 128
Streptococcus pneumoniae, 197
Streptococcus pyogenes, 14
Subarachnoid space, 189
Submandibular glands, ducts of, 190
Submucosa, 71
Succinyl-CoA, 70, 108
Sulphamethoxazole, 75
Sulphonamides, 32, 92
Superior gluteal artery, 175
Superior vena cava (SVC), 115
Suxamethonium, 16, 17

T

'Tailor's muscle,' 33
Takayasu arteritis, 39
Tardive dyskinesia, 52
TCA cycle, *see* Tricyclic acid cycle
T-cell receptor, 55
Temporal lobe, 12
Tendon, 58, 193
'Tennis elbow,' 95
Terminal ileum, 58
Testicular artery, 53
Tetracyclines, 91, 130
Tetrahydrofolic acid, 31
T4 (thyroxine), half-life of, 149
Thalassaemia, 92
Thiazide diuretics, 73
Thioureylenes, 13, 149
Thrombocyte, 14
Thromboxane A2, 131, 135, 147
Thyroid, 31, 94, 130
Thyroid-stimulating hormone (TSH), 130
Tidal volume, 172

Tirofiban, 174
Tissue plasminogen activator (t-PA), 96
T-lymphocytes (T-cells), 56, 89, 114, 171
TNF-α, *see* Tumour necrosis factor-α
Toll-like receptors (TLRs), 128
Tongue, anterior two-thirds of, 54
Total lung capacity, 172
Trabecular bone, 108
Trachea, C-shaped cartilaginous rings of, 56
Trachealis, 58
Tract of Goll, 71
Transfer RNA (tRNA), 147, 154
Transitional cell carcinoma, 169
Triceps brachii, 13
Tricuspid valve, 53–54
Tricyclic acid (TCA) cycle, 12, 72, 107
Tricyclic antidepressant, 19
Trigeminal nerve (CN V), 177
Trimethoprim, 31, 35, 75
Trochlear nerve, 191
Tropomyosin, 194, 197
Troponin, 194, 197
TSH, *see* Thyroid-stimulating hormone
Tuberculosis, 14, 35
Tumour necrosis factor-α (TNF-α),
        35, 38, 151
Turbinates, 192
Turner syndrome, 173
Type I alveolar cells, 134
Type I collagen, 113
Type II collagen, 51
Type III collagen, 150

U

Upper respiratory tract infections (URTIs), 75
Urine formation, 168
Uterus, 38

V

Vagal parasympathetic neurons, 15, 133
Vagus nerve (cranial nerve X), 16, 72, 193
Vascular endothelial growth factor (VEGF), 147
Vascular resistance, 91
Vasodilation, 148
Vasopressin, 94, 194
Ventricular repolarization, 172
Ventricular septal defects (VSDs), 176
Viral upper respiratory tract infections, 75
Vision, blurred, 18
Vital capacity (lung), 172
Vitamin B_{12}, 90, 93
Volkmann canals, 113
Voltage-gated Na^+ channels, 195

W

Warfarin, 148
Water (body), 95, 167
Wound contraction, 148, 149

X

Xanthopsia, 18
X-linked disorder, 111

Y

Yellow vision, 18

Z

Z-lines, 35
Zonula adherens, 53
Zonula occludens, 51
Zymogen, 167

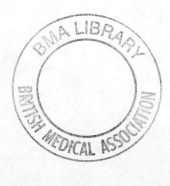